Speed, Ecstasy, Ritalin

Speed, Ecstasy, Ritalin

The Science of Amphetamines

LESLIE IVERSEN

Department of Pharmacology, University of Oxford

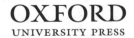

OXFORD
UNIVERSITY PRESS

Great Clarendon Street, Oxford OX2 6DP

Oxford University Press is a department of the University of Oxford.
It furthers the University's objective of excellence in research, scholarship,
and education by publishing worldwide in

Oxford New York

Auckland Cape Town Dar es Salaam Hong Kong Karachi
Kuala Lumpur Madrid Melbourne Mexico City Nairobi
New Delhi Shanghai Taipei Toronto

With offices in

Argentina Austria Brazil Chile Czech Republic France Greece
Guatemala Hungary Italy Japan Poland Portugal Singapore
South Korea Switzerland Thailand Turkey Ukraine Vietnam

Oxford is a registered trade mark of Oxford University Press
in the UK and in certain other countries

Published in the United States
by Oxford University Press Inc., New York

British Library Cataloguing in Publication Data

Data available

Library of Congress Cataloging in Publication Data

Iversen, Leslie L.
Speed, ecstasy, ritalin : the science of amphetamines / Leslie Iversen.
p. ; cm.
Includes bibliographical references and index.
1. Amphetamines. 2. Amphetamine abuse.
[DNLM: 1. Amphetamines—pharmacology. 2. Amphetamine-Related Disorders.
3. Amphetamines—therapeutic use. QV 102 194s 2006] I. Title.
HV5822.A5184 2006
616.86'4—dc22   2005036591

Typeset by Newgen Imaging Systems (P) Ltd., Chennai, India
Printed in Great Britain
on acid-free paper by
Biddles Ltd., King's Lynn

ISBN 0–19–853089–7 (Hbk)   978–0–19–853089–3 (Hbk: alk paper)

3 5 7 9 10 8 6 4 2

Contents

Acknowledgement

I would like to extend special thanks to Burt Angrist, one of the pioneers of amphetamine research, for his many helpful discussions and valuable information.

CHAPTER 1

Introduction

Amphetamines come in many different forms and have powerful effects for good and evil. An epidemic of methamphetamine abuse is currently sweeping through the USA and Southeast Asia; witness these stories from Hawaii, where the epidemic started in the 1980s, and from Thailand. In Hawaii:

> Twenty years old and fresh out of college Tad Yamaguchi saw a good future for himself at an air-freight company in Honolulu. So when one of his superiors offered him a puff from the small glass pipe—a little something to help him get through the gruelling 20 hour shift—Yamaguchi felt he couldn't refuse. He says he was instantly hooked. 'I felt alert, in control. It didn't seem to have a downside' recalls Yamaguchi. No wonder so many people in his office were using it. Four months later, Yamaguchi, who had never done drugs before, was smoking every day. 'I'd smoke as much as I could. I started buying large quantities to sell so I could support my habit' he says. Soon Yamaguchi, who kicked the habit a year ago, had lost 35 pounds and was smoking four days at a time, then 'crashing' in a comatose sleep that lasted up to 36 hours. Next paranoia and hallucinations set in. (M.A. Lerner, *Newsweek*, 27 November 1989)

And in Thailand:

> She has run out of methamphetamine, what the Thais call yaba (mad medicine), and she has become irritable and potentially violent. Jacky's cheeks are sunken, her skin pockmarked and her hair an unruly explosion of varying strands of red and brown. She is tall and skinny, and her arms and legs extend out from her narrow torso with its slightly protuberant belly like the appendages of a spider short-changed on legs.

> Sitting on the blue vinyl flooring of her Bangkok hut, Jacky leans her bare back against the plank wall, her dragon tattoos glistening with sweat as she trims her fingernails with a straight razor. It has been two days—no three—without sleep sitting in this hut and smoking the little pink speed tablets from sheets of tinfoil stripped from Krong Tip cigarette packets. Now as the flushes of artificial energy recede and the realization surfaces that there's no more money anywhere in her hut, Jacky is crashing hard, and she hates everyone and everything. (K.T. Greenfeld, Time, 2 April 2001)

Meanwhile another amphetamine-like chemical, methylphenidate (Ritalin) has proved popular for the treatment of children, and more recently adults, with attention deficit hyperactivity disorder (ADHD) on both sides of the Atlantic. Although the widespread use of this and related amphetamines in schoolchildren has raised much controversy, here is the story of one adult whose life was radically improved by Ritalin:

> I am a 35 year old male. Diagnosed with ADHD at 30 years of age. Exhibited classic, if not extreme symptoms of ADHD throughout my entire life. Currently on Wellbutrin SR for mild depression, and Ritalin SR for ADHD. I have exhibited absolutely no side effects from what is considered to be a fairly high dosage. (Ritalin SR 40 mg 2×/day). In fact I rarely experience any type of elevated heart rate and have the ability to fall asleep shortly after taking medication.

> According to those closest to me, I have undergone a transformation in my ability to pay attention and to communicate effectively. Relationships with family, friends, co-workers and customers have all flourished since I was diagnosed. It is very difficult to accurately describe my mental state when I am not on Ritalin. I can only say that I see the world through a fog that inhibits my ability to focus on external stimuli. Literally, I will find myself in a perpetual day dream. I could go on at length about the great challenges I was unable to overcome prior to my diagnosis. According to several doctors, because of a highly introspective personality, and being part of a very intelligent family, I intuitively made all of the changes recommended in one's lifestyle to overcome ADD/ADHD with or without the aid of psychostimulants. Because I had made these lifestyle changes, Ritalin was able to provide immediate and measurable results. Again, I need only ask those closest to me regarding these changes. Personally and professionally I have matured much more rapidly in these past five years than at any time in my life.

> Finally, I would like to address the raging debate over the over diagnosis of ADD, and the subsequent use of Ritalin and other stimulant medications. I tend to believe this is probably true. When combining our society's fast pace, with educational conformance, and the inability to definitively diagnosis those who truly have ADD/ADHD, we are bound to have misdiagnosis. Having said this, I am one of those extremely fortunate people who were correctly diagnosed. I have evolved over these past five years into a very happy and confident individual, and look forward to the future with great anticipation.

> I wish more people would share their success stories. It seems that those who are against Ritalin are by far the most outspoken. (http://neuro-www.mgh.harvard.edu/forum_2/ADHDF.html)

This book will seek to review the positive and negative aspects of amphetamines—man-made chemicals which had a great impact on the twentieth century and continue to do so in the new millennium. Benzedrine (DL-amphetamine) was introduced in the 1930s as a cold remedy to clear stuffy noses, but its medical uses multiplied and it enjoyed a brief vogue as a cure-all for many illnesses. For a while amphetamine and a variety of related chemicals found a huge market as appetite suppressants to counteract obesity, which became a preoccupation of twentieth-century life as Western societies prospered and hunger became largely a thing of the past. However, this part of the amphetamine story ended tragically with the introduction of an amphetamine combination treatment for obesity—the notorious 'phen-fen' mixture (phentermine plus fenfluramine) which led to thousands of premature deaths and heart damage and triggered the largest civil law suit ever seen. The pharmaceutical company responsible faced payments of more than $20 billion to claimants (see Chapter 3). There is still a large and growing medical use of amphetamines in the treatment of children suffering from attention-deficit hyperactivity disorder (ADHD), a market worth in excess of $2 billion annually. However, there has been controversy about the widespread use of these powerful drugs in schoolchildren. The scientific evidence for this and other medical uses of amphetamines will be examined in some detail

Almost as soon as Benzedrine first became available as a medicine many people found that they liked the psychostimulant effects that it produces. They felt more alert, had more energy, and could keep going at full speed for longer. Some liked the boost that the drug gives to sexual energy and fulfilment. The 'speed' drug fitted ideally into modern life with its 7-days-a-week 24-hours-a-day demands. However, what started as casual taking of amphetamines by students to help them prepare for examinations, or to improve stamina and endurance in sports activities (see Chapter 4), soon revealed a less benign face. Although it took a long time to be admitted fully, the fact is that amphetamines are potentially dangerous drugs of addiction. The modern versions of methamphetamine ('ice', 'crystal meth') which can be smoked or injected have proved particularly dangerous. The USA and parts of Southeast Asia are currently witnessing an alarming spread of methamphetamine abuse fuelled by plentiful supplies of the drug from small- and large-scale illicit manufacturers. It has proved all too easy to synthesize the drug from simple chemicals present in many cold-cure medicines (see Chapter 5).

The amphetamine-like drug ecstasy had its own impact on the social scene, becoming intimately associated with the 'rave dance' culture that flourished towards the end of the twentieth century. It too fitted the need for a chemical prop to facilitate social interactions and to give the participants energy to keep going all night long. It proved hugely popular, with millions of young people taking it each weekend, although the vogue may already be on the wane.

This book will tell some of these amphetamine stories in more detail from the perspective of a scientist who has undertaken basic research on how the amphetamines work in the brain and elsewhere in the body. This basic research paid considerable dividends; we now have a good understanding of the way in which amphetamines interact with naturally occurring chemical messengers, acting indirectly by stimulating release of these substances that are normally released only in response to nervous activity. An important by-product of this research was that it gave valuable clues about how the anti-psychotic drugs used to treat schizophrenia work in the brain, and lent support to the so-called 'dopamine hypothesis' of schizophrenia. High doses of amphetamines can lead to a temporary psychosis which resembles that of schizophrenia in many respects. The dopamine hypothesis proposes that both drug-induced and schizophrenic psychoses are due to an excessive release of the chemical messenger dopamine in the brain. Conversely, anti-psychotic drugs act by blocking the actions of dopamine.

More controversially, the evidence about just how dangerous amphetamines or ecstasy are will be reviewed dispassionately. Unfortunately, in their attempts to dissuade young people from taking these illegal drugs governments have tended to exaggerate their potential medical dangers. The author will take the view that ecstasy is a relatively safe drug which is not likely to cause irreversible brain damage. Its classification as a Schedule I (Category A) dangerous narcotic was almost certainly a mistake.

The illegal manufacture and sale of amphetamines has become a large and commercially valuable business. The first-ever United Nations global survey on ecstasy and amphetamines reported in September 2003 (United Nations 2003). It revealed a striking picture of increase in production and trafficking of these drugs. Seizures of amphetamines rose more than 10-fold in a period of 10 years, to almost 40 tonnes in 2000–2001. Estimated global production is more than 500 tonnes a year. It was estimated that, worldwide, 34 million people abuse amphetamine-like stimulants and 8 million use ecstasy. The business of illegal manufacture and supply of amphetamines and ecstasy was estimated to have an annual value of $65 billion, with profit margins as high as 3000–4000 per cent. Given these tempting returns and the ability to set up manufacture with relatively simple equipment, it is unlikely that this industry will be easy to shut down.

Despite the impact that amphetamines have had on human medicine and society, they have had remarkably little coverage. There have been some valuable books reviewing the subject, but they are relatively few and far between. The book *Speed Culture* (Grinspoon and Hedblom 1975) provided an excellent review of events up to 1975 and, more recently, Schliefer (1998) has reviewed the dangers of methamphetamine in the book *Methamphetamines: Speed Kills*. Sanello (2005) has described the devastating damage being done by methamphetamine in the gay community in America, and Choury and Meissonnier (2004) have reviewed the spread of methamphetamine abuse in Southeast Asia. Harris (2005) provides a collection of articles on the history and the contemporary amphetamine scene. It is hoped that the present volume will provide an additional objective account of some aspects of the uses and abuses of amphetamines.

CHAPTER 2

What are amphetamines and how do they work in the brain?

'In an effort to further our knowledge of the relationship between the chemical constitution and physiological action of compounds related to epinephrine and ephedrine, as well as to establish the possible therapeutic uses of phenylaminoethanol sulphate we have continued our investigation of this substance.'

(Piness *et al.* 1930)

2.1. Chemistry

The amphetamines are man-made chemicals which bear a close resemblance to a number of naturally occurring substances. Phenylethylamine (Fig. 2.1), for example, is found in many foodstuffs, particularly cheeses and some wines. It is taken into the body in the diet but has little or no effect because it is rapidly degraded as it passes in the blood from the digestive system to the liver where it is degraded by the enzyme monoamine oxidase, together with other related dietary amines that might otherwise have hazardous effects in the body. Amphetamine is a simple synthetic derivative of phenylethylamine which differs only in possessing a methyl group ($-CH_3$) attached to the side chain. However, this is a very significant alteration as the methyl group protects amphetamine from degradation by monoamine oxidase, and hence the man-made drug, which exerts a variety of biological effects, can enter and persist in the bloodstream.

Because the methyl group of amphetamine can be attached to the side chain in a left- or right-handed manner, amphetamine exists in two different mirror-image forms, or stereoisomers. One of these, the right-handed or dextro-isomer, is far more biologically active than the left-handed or levo-isomer. It is referred to as 'D-amphetamine' (also S(+)amphetamine, dexamphetamine, dexedrine). There are many different variants of the basic chemical structure of amphetamine, some of which are illustrated in Figure 2.1. For example, addition of a second methyl group to the basic nitrogen of the side chain leads to methamphetamine which has even more potent biological actions. Again, the dextro-isomer is the more powerful. Further chemical alterations to the benzene ring

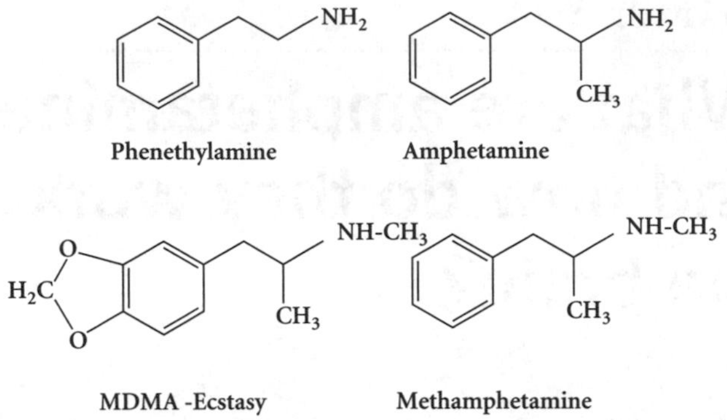

Phenethylamine   Amphetamine

MDMA -Ecstasy   Methamphetamine

Figure 2.1 Similarities between amphetamines, the natural product phenethylamine, and ecstasy.

lead to methylene-dioxy-methamphetamine (MDMA) commonly known as 'ecstasy'. These are only a few examples of an almost unlimited number of chemical variations that can be made on this basic scaffold. The American chemists Alexander and Ann Shulgin have described 179 different synthetic phenylethylamines which they made and tested for their psychic effects, using mainly themselves as guinea pigs. Their results are described in the remarkable book *Pihkal* (phenylethylamines I have known and loved) (Shulgin and Shulgin 2000). Although the Shulgins made a unique and valuable contribution to knowledge in this field, their activities were always just one step ahead of the law, and the US authorities finally forced them to close their laboratory. Pharmaceutical companies also discovered a variety of compounds with somewhat more complex chemical structures which act by the same mechanism as the classical amphetamines; some examples are illustrated in Figure 2.2.

In addition to the man-made amphetamines and related compounds there is one naturally occurring compound which closely resembles the amphetamines chemically and which shares the same pharmacology. This is cathinone (Fig. 2.3), the principal active ingredient in the khat shrub whose leaves have been chewed by the peoples of East Africa and the Arab Peninsula for their psychostimulant properties for many hundreds of years (see Chapter 5).

2.2. How are amphetamines administered?

In order to be easily administered drugs should be soluble in water, but in order to penetrate into the brain they must pass the 'blood–brain barrier' which protects the brain from dietary toxins. To cross this barrier some degree of solubility in fat is required. The amphetamines have almost the ideal combination of water and fat solubility. This means that they are easily administered by a variety of routes and they penetrate readily and rapidly into the central nervous system (CNS).

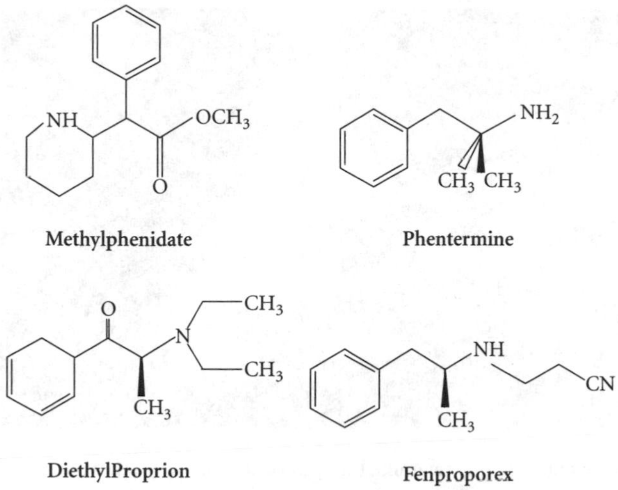
NH
OCH3
O
Methylphenidate
NH2
CH3 CH3
Phentermine
O
CH3
N
CH3
CH3
DiethylProprion
NH
CN
CH3
Fenproporex

Figure 2.2 Man-made amphetamine-like drugs. All of these are approved medicines used as appetite suppressants for the treatment of obesity or for treating ADHD in children.

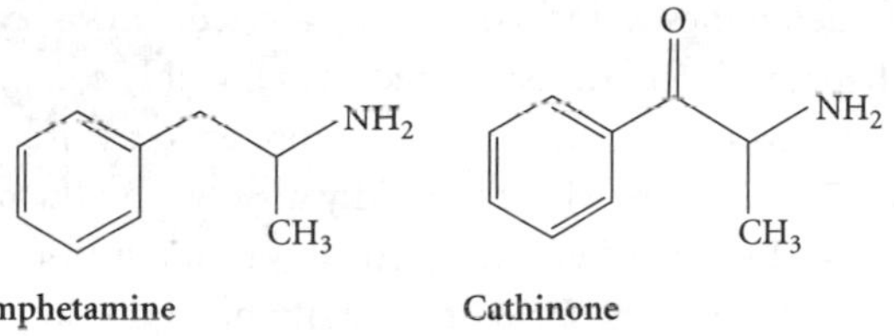
NH2
CH3
Amphetamine
O
NH2
CH3
Cathinone

Figure 2.3 Similarities between amphetamine structure and that of cathinone.

However, pure amphetamines are organic amines which exist as oily liquids that are not very soluble in water. This problem is overcome by preparing an acid salt form by neutralizing the organic base with an acid. The salts most commonly used are amphetamine sulphate and methamphetamine hydrochloride. These are white crystalline solids which are freely soluble in water. Once in the body, the salt dissociates to release the free amine form of the drug which is the active form.

Amphetamine salts can be administered in a variety of ways. For medical or military use, the compound is taken by mouth as a tablet or capsule containing a carefully measured dose. The drug dissolves in the stomach and is gradually absorbed as it passes through the gut. This method of administration provides a gradual absorption of drug and a prolonged duration of action. This avoids a rapid peak of drug level in the blood which could cause excessive psychostimulant effects.

However, it is precisely such effects that the amphetamine addict craves. When the drugs are abused they are usually administered by a method that

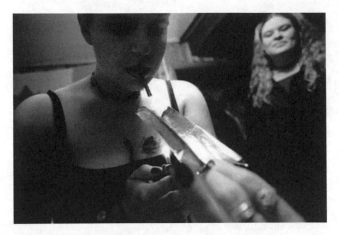

Figure 2.4 Smoking methamphetamine hydrochloride ('ice', 'crystal meth').

ensures rapid absorption and almost instant delivery to the brain. An obvious way of achieving this is to inject a solution containing the drug into a vein, and this is how amphetamines were traditionally abused. Nowadays, with the danger of HIV or hepatitis infection associated with possibly contaminated needles, injection is a less favoured route. Users may prefer to insufflate the powdered drug by sniffing into the nose where it rapidly dissolves on the nasal membranes and is quickly absorbed. An alternative, which was first introduced in Hawaii in the 1980s (Cho 1990), uses the form of methamphetamine known as 'ice' which can be smoked after heating in a small glass pipe or on a piece of aluminium foil (Fig. 2.4). Smoking delivers the drug to the extensive surface area of membranes in the lung where it is rapidly absorbed. 'Ice' or 'crystal meth' is a specially prepared form of pure D-methamphetamine hydrochloride which is translucent and resembles rock candy. The common salt form of D-amphetamine is amphetamine sulphate, which has a very high melting point (300°C). This makes it impossible to smoke, since heating above 300°C causes chemical decomposition. The melting point of D-methamphetamine hydrochloride (172 °C) is sufficiently low to allow vaporization without decomposition on smoking.

The majority of ecstasy users take the drug as a tablet by mouth, although it can also be insufflated or injected. Ecstasy users presumably want the drug to have a prolonged action as it helps to keep them awake for the all-night dance scene with which it is often associated.

All the amphetamines are readily absorbed into the bloodstream from the various routes of administration, where they persist for long periods of time. Half-lives for elimination from the blood are in the range of 6–12 hours. D-Methamphetamine has a particularly long half-life of 11–12 hours.

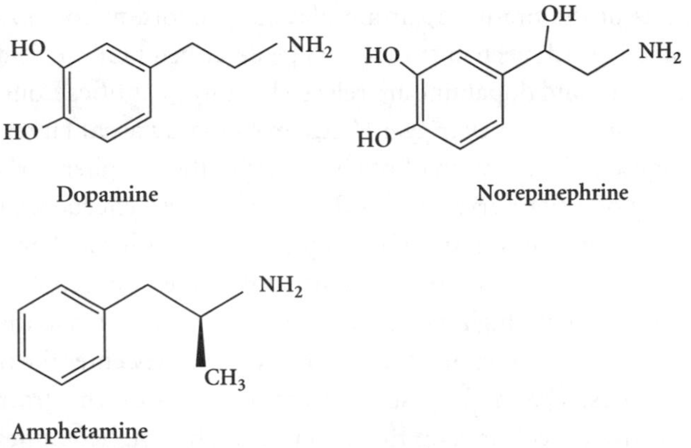

Dopamine

Norepinephrine

Amphetamine

Figure 2.5 Amphetamine structure resembles that of the naturally occurring neurotransmitters dopamine and norepinephrine.

2.3. How do amphetamines work?

The amphetamines are chemically related to the naturally occurring catecholamine neurotransmitter substances norepinephrine and dopamine (Fig. 2.5). These are among the many chemical messenger molecules used by nerves to activate target organs or for nerve cells in the brain to communicate with each other (reviewed by Iversen 2001).

Despite the close chemical resemblance to the naturally occurring neurotransmitters, amphetamines are not able to activate the cellular receptors normally stimulated by norepinephrine or dopamine. Instead, they act by stimulating the release of these natural neurotransmitters. In peripheral tissues amphetamine stimulates the release of norepinephrine from the nerve endings of the 'sympathetic nervous system' which controls a variety of peripheral functions (see section 2.4). Because of its ability to stimulate functions normally controlled by the sympathetic nervous system, amphetamine has long been recognized as a 'sympathomimetic amine' (Trendelenburg 1963).

There are also nerve cells in the brain which store and release norepinephrine; these play a variety of roles, for example in helping to alert the higher centres in the brain to interesting events in the outside world and helping in the laying down of new memories. The closely related substance dopamine is an intermediate in the biosynthesis of norepinephrine, but also acts in its own right as a chemical messenger, found almost exclusively in the brain. Dopamine is present in different types of nerve cells from those containing norepinephrine. It also has a number of different roles. The release of dopamine in a part of the brain known as the 'basal ganglia' plays a vital role in the control of voluntary movements. Patients with Parkinson's disease have a selective loss of dopamine-containing cells from the brain, and they find it difficult to initiate movement.

In other parts of the brain dopamine plays an important role in emotional behaviour and reward mechanisms, as will be described in more detail below.

Norepinephrine and dopamine are released in tiny quantities from the nerves which contain them and they trigger effects in closely adjacent target cells (contraction of muscle or activation of other targets in the periphery, or changes in the excitability of other nerve cells in the brain). These effects occur after the chemical messengers bind to specific receptor molecules located on the surface of the target cells. These receptors recognize dopamine or norepinephrine with great sensitivity and are highly selective. Amphetamines activate the receptors for dopamine and norepinephrine indirectly because they enter the nerves containing these substances and cause a release of the natural neurotransmitter, which then activates receptors on the target cells. The amphetamines can enter the dopamine- or norepinephrine-containing nerve partly because they are sufficiently lipid soluble to cross the nerve cell membrane (Mack and Bonisch 1979; Liang and Rutledge 1982). However, more importantly, amphetamines are also selectively concentrated in norepinephrine- and dopamine-containing nerves because they are pumped in by the transporter molecules that normally help to remove and recapture the neurotransmitters after their release (Fig. 2.6). Once inside the nerve cell, the amphetamines are recognized by the separate transporter mechanism which helps to concentrate the natural neurotransmitters inside storage vesicles in the nerve terminals (Fig. 2.6). Mobilizing stored neurotransmitter from these storage vesicles causes accumulation of an unusually high concentration of neurotransmitter in the cytoplasm, and this may be amplified by the additional property of amphetamine to act as an inhibitor of the enzyme monoamine oxidase which acts to degrade free intracellular monoamines. The increased level of free catecholamine in the cytoplasm leads, in turn, to a release of neurotransmitter as the transporter mechanism works in reverse to remove neurotransmitter from the nerve terminal. A continuing inflow of amphetamine via the transporter may facilitate a 'counter-transport' of dopamine outwards, as it makes the substrate binding site of the transporter more frequently available at the inner surface of the nerve cell membrane. A study of the details of amphetamine action by means of electrical recordings of currents across fragments of dopamine membrane from dopamine nerve cells showed that amphetamine can also trigger brief pulses of rapid dopamine release, resembling those seen during the normal neurotransmitter release process (Kahlig et al. 2005). The importance of the actions of amphetamine on the vesicular transporter versus the cell membrane transporters remains unclear (Jones et al. 1998; Fleckenstein et al. 2000; Rothman and Baumann 2003). However, an action on the cell membrane transporter appears to be critical. Brain slices prepared from mice that were genetically engineered so that they did not express the dopamine transporter (DAT knockout) failed to show any

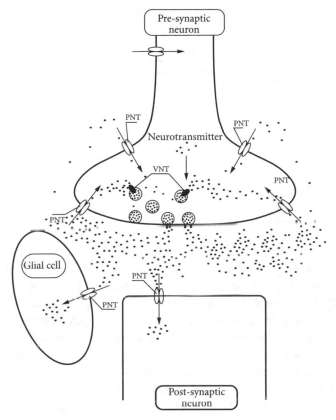

Figure 2.6 Role of plasma membrane neurotransmitter transporters (PNTs) and vesicle neurotransmitter transporter (VNTs) in the storage and inactivation of neurotransmitters. (Redrawn from J. Masson *et al.*, *Pharmacol Rev*, **51**, 439–464, 1999.)

increase in dopamine release when amphetamine was added to the incubating fluid, whereas this was readily demonstrated in brain slices prepared from normal mice (Jones *et al.* 1998). These authors also showed that administration of a high dose of amphetamine (10 mg/kg interperitoneally) to DAT knockout mice failed to cause the normal burst of dopamine release seen in the dopamine-rich basal ganglia region of brain. These experiments involved the implantation in the mouse brain of fine electrodes designed to detect the released dopamine.

Amphetamine and methamphetamine are recognized almost equally well by the norepinephrine and dopamine transporters and they cause release of both these neurotransmitters (Table 2.1). In the brain, however, they appear to be more effective in releasing dopamine than norepinephrine. In the intact rat brain a release of norepinephrine can also be measured in response to

Table 2.1 Affinities of monoamines and amphetamines at monoamine transporters in rat brain

Compound	K_i (nM)		
	Norepinephrine	Serotonin	Dopamine
Dopamine	40	6489	38
Norepinephrine	64	>50,000	357
Serotonin	3013	17	2703
D-Amphetamine	39	3830	35
D-Methamphetamine	48	2137	114
Ecstasy (MDMA)	462	238	1572

K_i, nanomolar concentration needed to occupy half of the monoamine transporter sites.
Data from Rothman and Baumann 2003.

amphetamine (Kuczenski and Segal 1992), but it has proved more difficult to demonstrate drug-induced norepinephrine release *in vitro* (Kuczenski and Segal 1992). It is possible that amphetamine is less effective in mobilizing norepinephrine from vesicle stores than dopamine, and such mobilization may be necessary for a robust response (Trendelenburg 1991). Overall, there is little change in the metabolic turnover of norepinephrine in rat brain (a measure of the rate of monoamine synthesis, release, and degradation) in response to amphetamine, whereas there is an increased turnover of dopamine (Costa *et al.* 1972). It seems that it is the ability of amphetamines to stimulate dopamine release in the brain that explains most, if not all, of their psychostimulant properties.

Ecstasy (MDMA) is an unusual member of the amphetamine family as it has some ability to release dopamine and norepinephrine, but has a higher affinity for the transporter in serotonin (5-HT) neurons; thus its main effect is to promote an increased release of serotonin in the brain (Table 2.1).

2.4. Peripheral effects of amphetamines

Amphetamines not only cause a release of monoamine neurotransmitters in the brain, but also stimulate the release of norepinephrine from nerve terminals of the sympathetic nervous system in the periphery. The sympathetic nervous system is involved in the reflex control of a variety of bodily functions, regulating the strength and rate of heart beat, blood pressure, gut movements, and various glandular functions. The terminals of sympathetic nerves release norepinephrine as their principal neurotransmitter. Amphetamines interact with the norepinephrine transporter and storage vesicle mechanisms in these nerve terminals to cause a release of norepinephrine that is independent of nerve activity (Trendelenburg 1963). In practice this means that amphetamines cause an increase in blood pressure and pulse rate in both animals and humans. At high doses of amphetamine the effect may be mainly on blood pressure, as the heart automatically compensates for large increases in blood pressure by slowing down (Peoples and Guttmann 1936; Altschule and Iglauer 1940; Schindler *et al.* 1992). The effects on blood pressure are mediated by norepinephrine acting on α-adrenoceptors on blood vessels to constrict them; the effects on the heart involve the action of norepinephrine on β-adrenoceptors on heart muscle. Part of the cardiovascular action may also be due to a release of dopamine (Schindler *et al.* 1992). Other sympathomimetic effects include dry mouth, retention of urine, and sometimes increased respiratory rate.

Some of the sympathomimetic effects of amphetamine can have medical benefits. In the lung the effect of amphetamine-induced norepinephrine release is to dilate the airways and make breathing easier for asthma sufferers; this was one of the earliest medical uses of these drugs (see Chapter 3). Amphetamine was also used initially as a nasal decongestant because of its ability to cause norepinephrine release which constricts the blood vessels in the nasal cavity and reduces the increased blood flow and inflammation which accompany a cold.

The peripheral effects of the amphetamines, especially the increased pulse, are subjectively obvious to the drug user. They are also potentially life-threatening. Most of the amphetamine-related deaths reported each year are due to excessive stimulation of heart and blood pressure, leading to stroke (damage and bleeding in blood vessels in the brain) or heart failure (cf Chapter 7). Chronic amphetamine users can develop irregular heart beat as well as inflammation and damage to the heart (Yu *et al.* 2003). The peripheral cardiovascular effects of amphetamines set a limit to the psychostimulant dose that can safely be used. In this respect D-methamphetamine has a slightly higher safety window than D-amphetamine; the two drugs have about the same potency as sympathomimetics, but D-methamphetamine is at least twice as potent as a central nervous system stimulant. This may partly explain the ever-increasing popularity of D-methamphetamine as a drug of abuse.

2.5. Psychostimulant effects of amphetamines in animals

Amphetamines have a number of easily observed effects on animal behaviour and these have been extensively studied in order to understand the underlying brain mechanisms. The most frequently used species are rats and mice. Low doses of D-amphetamine (0.1–1.0 mg/kg) cause a dose-dependent stimulation of activity in these animals, and higher doses can lead to prolonged running activity. This is easily quantified in automated activity cages and provides a simple model system. The response is particularly notable since the tests are normally carried out during the day when rodents, which are nocturnal animals, are not normally very active.

Higher doses of D-amphetamine (5–10 mg/kg) cause an entirely different pattern of behaviour in animals, characterized by the continuous repetition of purposeless movements referred to as 'stereotyped behaviour' (Randrup and Munkvad 1974; Wallach 1974). The pattern of movements is characteristic for different species. In rodents, stereotyped behaviour normally consists of continuous head-swaying, sniffing, licking, and gnawing. Instead of the purposeful running activity seen after lower doses of the drug, animals exhibiting stereotyped behaviour will often stay in one part of the cage and continuously repeat these behaviours. After administering a high dose of amphetamine there is a period of intense stereotypy, followed by running activity as the drug level in the blood gradually falls as the drug is metabolized and excreted. Stereotyped behaviour can also be elicited by high doses of D-amphetamine in monkeys where behaviour is more varied but generally includes repetitive movements of the head, tongue, lips, hands, and arms.

An unusual feature of the behavioural response to amphetamine is that they show 'sensitization' on repeated administration of the drug. Thus repeated daily administration of amphetamine gradually leads to exaggerated running and stereotypy responses, and this effect persists for some days after repeat administration is stopped (Segal and Kuczenski 1996). The mechanisms underlying the behavioural sensitization to amphetamine remain unclear. Several studies have reported increased amphetamine-induced release of dopamine in various brain regions in sensitized animals, and have proposed a variety of explanations for this (reviewed by Segal and Kuczinski 1996). However, others found that behavioural sensitization can also occur even when the amount of dopamine released is normal or even decreased below normal (Guix et al. 1992; Segal and Kuczenski 1992). Although behavioural responses to amphetamine appear to be triggered by a release of dopamine in the brain, the behavioural and neurochemical responses are not linked together quantitatively in any simple manner. Measurements of amphetamine-induced dopamine release in the intact brain have shown that while the time course of dopamine release parallels the appearance and disappearance of amphetamine in the bloodstream, the behavioural responses often persist for much longer. Rats may continue to exhibit stereotypy long after the rate of dopamine release has dropped below its peak (Segal and Kuczenski 1996). Seeman et al. (2005) suggested that sensitization might be caused by a persistent shift in the sensitivity of dopamine D_2 receptors in brain to dopamine. They showed by radioligand binding studies that in animals sensitized by repeated treatment with amphetamine a higher proportion of the D_2 receptors in brain were of a higher affinity subtype than previously.

A series of experiments led to the conclusion that all these psychostimulant effects of D-amphetamine can be attributed to its ability to release dopamine in the brain. Studies in the 1960s and 1970s showed that the behavioural effects of

D-amphetamine could be completely blocked by treating animals beforehand with the compound α-methyl tyrosine, which inhibits the biosynthesis of catecholamines and leads to a depletion of the brain stores (Weissman *et al.* 1966; Thornburg and Moore 1973). However, this compound blocks the synthesis of both dopamine and norepinephrine, and so the result did not indicate which was the more important. Thornburg and Moore used an inhibitor of the enzyme dopamine-β-hydroxylase, which catalyses the last step in norepinephrine biosynthesis from dopamine. This treatment, which selectively depleted norepinephrine but not dopamine, failed to block the behavioural stimulant effects of D-amphetamine, suggesting that it is drug-induced dopamine release which is the key factor.

It was also found that classical anti-psychotic drugs ('neuroleptics') of many different chemical types (e.g. chlorpromazine, haloperidol) were effective antagonists of both the running activity and stereotyped behaviour responses elicited by D-amphetamine in rodents (Janssen *et al.* 1965). Indeed, this finding was so consistent that the ability of compounds to block the stimulant actions of amphetamine became one of the standard tests used to screen for new anti-schizophrenic drugs (see Chapter 6). Although it was not known in the 1960s, we now understand that all drugs in this class act as antagonists at dopamine receptors in the brain (Creese *et al.* 1976a,b).

Further insight into the importance of the dopamine neurons in the brain in mediating the various behavioural responses to D-amphetamine was provided by experiments in which these neurons were selectively destroyed in different brain regions. The compound 6-hydroxydopamine is an analogue of dopamine which is selectively taken up and accumulated by the transporters in norepinephrine- and dopamine-containing neurons. Once inside the neurons, the compound causes a series of toxic chemical reactions which lead to the permanent destruction of the neurons. 6-Hydroxydopamine cannot penetrate into the brain from the bloodstream and so it has to be administered directly by micro-injection into brain. By using very small doses administered into precise anatomical locations it is possible to create selective damage to particular groups of norepinephrine- or dopamine-containing neurons. Selective lesions of norepinephrine neurons were found to have little effect on the stimulant actions of D-amphetamine, but the stimulant actions were completely absent in animals with selective dopamine lesions (Creese and Iversen 1974; Hollister *et al.* 1974).

Further studies with 6-hydroxydopamine showed that different groups of dopamine neurons in brain are responsible for the stimulant (running activity) and stereotyped behaviour responses to D-amphetamine. In rats in which the dopamine stores in the basal ganglia were destroyed by local micro-injections of 6-hydroxydopamine, the stereotyped behaviour response to high doses of

D-amphetamine were greatly reduced, while the running response remained intact (Price and Fibiger 1974; Kelly *et al.* 1975). The latter authors went on to show that micro-injections of 6-hydroxydopamine into the nucleus accumbens (a dopamine-rich region located deep in the forebrain and part of a separate dopamine-containing neural pathway) abolished the running response to D-amphetamine while leaving the stereotyped behaviour response intact, suggesting that dopamine release in different brain regions mediates different elements of the behavioural response.

Another experimental approach which has yielded valuable insights into the effects of amphetamine and other drugs has been the drug-discrimination procedure (Brauer *et al.* 1997). In this paradigm animals are trained to discriminate between two substances they have received (usually test drug versus saline); by pressing the 'drug' lever in the test cage on receiving the drug the animal gains a food reward. Rats learn quite readily to distinguish even very small doses of D-amphetamine or related drugs from saline. Animals trained in this way can provide a wealth of valuable information. Although the animal cannot describe the overall subjective effect of the drug, it can be asked to tell the experimenter whether the effect of one amphetamine is different from another. For example, rats trained to recognize D-amphetamine cannot tell the difference if methamphetamine, methylphenidate, or other related amphetamine-like drugs are substituted, but they will not generalize to MDMA or fenfluramine, which are amphetamine derivatives that act predominantly via a serotoninergic rather than a dopaminergic mechanism. We can also ask which of the several different types of dopamine receptor in the brain are most important in mediating the amphetamine cue. Drugs that act as direct stimulants at dopamine D_2 receptors (e.g. quinpirole, pergolide) are good substitutes for D-amphetamine, but drugs that act on dopamine D_1 or D_3 receptors are not. As expected, antagonist drugs that block dopamine actions at D_2 receptors also abolish the animals' ability to discriminate D-amphetamine from saline. It is even possible to ask which regions of brain are most important for the dopamine-mediated amphetamine cue. Rats recognized direct micro-injections of dopamine into areas of the frontal-brain mesolimbic system as a drug cue, whereas injections into the striatum, another dopamine-rich brain region, were not recognized in this way (reviewed by Brauer *et al.* 1997).

Other neurotransmitters in brain interact with the primary dopamine mechanism triggered by D-amphetamine. Thus, for example, while D-amphetamine has little ability to directly stimulate serotonin release from brain (Chiueh and Moore 1976), the serotonin system in brain appears to act as a brake on dopamine-mediated responses. Treatment of rats with drugs that inhibit the biosynthesis of serotonin (e.g. *p*-chlorophenylalanine) or selective serotonin neurotoxins(e.g. 5,6-dihyroxytryptamine) lead to exaggerated behavioural responses to D-amphetamine (Mabry and Campbell 1973; Breese *et al.* 1974). Acetylcholine-containing neurons in brain also seem to interact antagonistically with dopamine neurons. Treatment with drugs which block acetylcholine receptors enhanced behavioural responses to D-amphetamine (Arnfred and Randrup 1968; Carlton 1968), whereas drugs that activate acetylcholine receptors diminished D-amphetamine responses (Mennear 1965; Arnfred and Randrup 1968).

2.6. Effects of amphetamines on human mood and performance

While studies of amphetamine responses in animals have given us important insights into the brain mechanisms involved, studies of the effects of amphetamines on the human brain show how complex the effects of these drugs are. There is an extensive human literature describing the effects of these drugs. Probably the first discovery of the psychostimulant effects of amphetamine was made by the British chemist Gordon Alles, who synthesized and tested the compound on animals and on himself (Alles 1928). He quickly discovered that amphetamine powerfully alleviated fatigue and created euphoric confidence and alertness. One of the first attempts at a scientific study was made in 1935 by M. H. Nathanson, a Los Angeles physician who studied the subjective effects of amphetamine in 55 young hospital workers who were each given 20 mg of Benzedrine (the mixture of D- and L-amphetamine available at that time) (Nathanson 1937). The two most commonly reported drug effects were 'a sense of well being and a feeling of exhilaration' and 'lessened fatigue in reaction to work'. Some of the phrases used were as follows (Grinspoon and Hedblom 1975):

> 'increased energy, felt as I could not get places fast enough'; 'I have done things today I usually dislike but which I rather enjoyed doing today'; 'the last hour and a half of work is usually an effort, today I felt fine'; 'did not have my usual lethargic period after lunch'; 'sense of well being, nothing seemed impossible of accomplishment'; 'I wanted to stop and talk to everybody I met'; 'I felt unusually friendly towards other people'; 'my spirits have been high all day, felt bubbling inside'; 'I was able to organize my work quickly and efficiently'; 'my mind felt clear all day'.

A similar study carried out on 100 volunteers in Denmark came to the same conclusions (Bahnsen *et al.* 1938). The researchers were impressed by the large number of subjects who said that amphetamine increased their desire for work, or made them feel that it was easier to get started or to perform a task. Many subjects reported enhanced general well-being, good humour, loquaciousness, excitement, and exhilaration. Very few reported adverse psychic effects, although there were some 'organic symptoms', presumably related to actions on the peripheral sympathetic nervous system, including dry mouth, palpitations, headache, and muscle weakness. Several subjects reported disturbed sleep and decreased appetite.

The powerful euphoriant effects of amphetamine were also clear in a study in which amphetamine was compared with morphine and heroin in a group of 20 volunteers (Lasagna *et al.* 1955). The drugs were administered under double-blind conditions (i.e. neither the subject nor the doctor knew which drug was being given). Heroin and morphine proved to have little appeal. After low doses of heroin, only neutral or unpleasant reactions were reported; after higher doses, most subjects found it unpleasant with only two finding it pleasant. Reactions to morphine were even more negative; half of the subjects taking the higher dose considered it the most unpleasant medicine in the series and only two found it pleasant. These findings tally with the experience of doctors who use these drugs to treat pain in the clinic; very few patients experience euphoria and the idea that the medical use of a single dose of heroin can create an addict is simply an unfortunate myth. Reactions of the same subjects to amphetamine were in marked contrast. Thirteen of the 20 subjects rated it the most enjoyable of all drugs tested. Fourteen wanted to take it again. Among the comments made were the following (Grinspoon and Hedblom 1975):

> JC: The most striking effect occurred very soon after medication. Suddenly my body felt light and I became very happy, indeed exhilarated. This new state filled me with excitement and joy. A delightful drug!

> PL: An 'all over' good feeling. I felt capable of doing almost any task (within reason; at least I felt I could make a darned good try at accomplishing almost any task), and I felt confident of my abilities, not only for the present time, but also for the future . . . The drug is a good 'pick-me-up'.

> HM: The medication took no effect for perhaps ten minutes. Then I began to feel a deep sense of well being come over me and a feeling of control over myself and confidence and power. I feel similar when I'm playing the piano at my best . . . a feeling of exhilaration and satisfaction, not unlike the feeling that accompanies sexual satisfaction. All feelings of inadequacy or depression that I've felt at other times seem remote and trivial.

These are typical of the effects of relatively low doses of amphetamine in normal healthy people. With somewhat larger doses (in the range 20–50 mg D-amphetamine) all these effects are intensified, but the feeling of 'relaxed alertness' is replaced by a 'driven' feeling. Thoughts cascade rapidly through the mind and the capacity to concentrate is diminished. A sense of earnestness and decreased frivolity are often felt, and the user may feel compelled to bore others with increased talkativeness about serious or inappropriate subjects.

However, these relatively benign effects of orally administered amphetamine are not what the addict craves. Amphetamine abusers use high doses of the drug taken intravenously or by some other means that ensures rapid delivery to the bloodstream and brain (smoking, insufflation). The resulting 'rush' is a far more intense experience. The 'rush' or 'flash', as the initial experience is called, is an event much prized by the addict. It has been described by Rylander (1969) as follows:

> One of the addicts. . . . said that at first he feels numbed and if he is standing he goes down on his knees. The heart starts beating at a terrible speed and his respiration is very rapid. Then he feels as if he is ascending into the cosmos, every fibre of his body trembling with happiness.

The intensity of the 'rush' is dose related and this often leads addicts to increase the drug dosage. Moreover, the desire to repeat the experience can lead the addict into a cycle of repeated and increasing dosage. This in turn can result in periods of unproductive frenzied activity, stereotyped behaviour, and even psychosis (see Chapter 6), alternating with exhaustion, extended sleep, profound depression of mood, and lethargy (Angrist and Sudilovsky 1978). Similar patterns of repeated cycles of amphetamine intake have been observed in rats or monkeys in experiments in which the animals were able to self-administer the drug by intravenous injection (Schuster et al. 1969; Pickens et al. 1972).

As in the animal experiments, all the psychostimulant effects of amphetamine in humans are believed to be due to its ability to release dopamine in the brain. In support of this, as in animals, the catecholamine biosynthesis inhibitor α-methyl-tyrosine was found to be an effective antagonist of the human stimulant response to D-amphetamine (Jönsson et al. 1969, 1971). However, it has proved more difficult to show that the euphoriant and stimulant effects of amphetamine are blocked by drugs which act as antagonists at dopamine receptors in the brain. Early studies in regular users of amphetamine showed an attenuation of the euphoric and stimulant effects following administration of the anti-schizophrenic drugs pimozide and chlorpromazine (Gunne et al. 1972; Jönsson 1972), but subsequent studies in normal volunteers have generally yielded negative or equivocal data (reviewed by Brauer et al. 1997). One problem is that the doses of the antagonist drugs normally used clinically in the treatment of schizophrenia do not achieve a complete blockade of dopamine D_2 receptors in the brain. Independent brain imaging studies suggest that, at best, these drugs achieve only 60–80 per cent occupancy of the dopamine receptors. This may not be enough to counteract the powerful amphetamine-induced wave of dopamine release in brain. The use of higher doses in human studies is ruled out by ethical considerations because of the unpleasant and potentially serious side effects seen after high doses of such drugs as pimozide or chlorpromazine.

As with most other psychoactive drugs, there is considerable variability in individual responses to amphetamines. Not everyone finds their effects pleasant; some experience little subjective response at all, while others find that amphetamine provokes anxiety rather than euphoria. Some of the underlying neurobiological reasons for such individual differences are beginning to be understood, and genetic differences play an important part. Lott *et al.* (2005) studied responses to two doses of D-amphetamine (10 and 20 mg) versus placebo in 101 healthy young male and female volunteers. Blood samples taken for DNA analysis focused on minor genetically determined variants in the gene coding for the dopamine transporter protein. It was found that those people who possessed two copies (one from each parent) of the '9-repeat' version of the gene experienced virtually no subjective responses to the drug, in terms of either euphoria or anxiety. This version of the gene is also known to result in lower levels of expression of the dopamine transporter protein, a key target of amphetamine's effects. Stein *et al.* (2002) have previously reported that children who have the '9-repeat' version of the dopamine transporter gene show blunted responses to the amphetamine-like stimulant methylphenidate (see Chapter 3). Volkow *et al.* (2003) reported that people who found amphetamine pleasant tended to have lower levels of dopamine D_2 receptors in their brains (assessed by positron-emission tomography imaging techniques), suggesting the possibility that their brain dopamine system could benefit most from a drug-induced 'boost'.

Hormonal factors can also influence subjective responsiveness to amphetamine. White *et al.* (2002) studied 13 normal healthy women at different stages of the menstrual cycle, and found that positive subjective responses to 15 mg D-amphetamine administered orally were significantly higher during the follicular phase of the cycle than during the luteal phase, and that the responsiveness in the follicular phase showed a positive correlation with levels of the female hormone oestradiol.

As in the animal drug-discrimination studies described above, human subjects can learn to discriminate the 'amphetamine cue' from placebo (Kamien *et al.* 1993; Brauer *et al.* 1997). The latter authors showed that when people were trained to recognize D-amphetamine, other amphetamines were able to substitute fully (i.e. the subjects could not tell the difference) but higher doses were required, with the following potency ratios: phenmetrazine, 2.5; phenyl-propanolamine, (norephedrine), 7.5; methylphenidate, 2.0. These drugs are all capable of mimicking the dopamine-releasing effect of D-amphetamine. In contrast, fenfluramine, which acts predominantly via serotonin release, substituted only partially for D-amphetamine as a drug cue (Kamien *et al.* 1993).

2.7. Effects on cognitive performance

One of the most common reasons cited by students, truck drivers, soldiers, or businessmen for taking amphetamines is that they enhance performance and stave off normal fatigue. A considerable experimental literature in animals and in human subjects has sought to document this.

In animal models of learning and memory it is not always easy to demonstrate an enhancement of performance with drugs. Animals may be highly trained to undertake simple and more complex tasks, for example rats trained to press a lever to obtain food rewards and then required to discriminate different visual signals or to remember them in order to know the 'correct' lever response. However, the performance of highly trained animals is near perfect with very few errors, and so drugs cannot improve it further. What low doses of amphetamine consistently do is to speed up performance, so that reaction times are shortened and latencies to respond decrease (reviewed by Grilly and Loveland 2001). This often occurs without any loss of accuracy. The performance-enhancing effects of amphetamine are most apparent in tasks that require sustained attention.

In some tests speeded-up responses can lead to errors. Robbins (2002) reviewed results from one widely used test of accuracy and attention: the five-choice serial reaction time task. In this test rats face a series of adjacent apertures, each of which can contain an illuminated cue. The animal has to react within 5 seconds of the light going off by poking its nose into the aperture to trigger an infrared switch. The test continues for up to 100 trials, with correct responses rewarded by food pellets. An accuracy of around 80 per cent is readily achieved in well-trained rats, leaving little room for drug-induced improvement. Indeed, performance after administration of amphetamine tended to become worse because animals responded prematurely, and responses in an inter-trial interval of 5 seconds were punished by a 5 second lights-out period. However, animals who exhibited poor baseline accuracy in this test did respond positively to low doses of the amphetamine analogue methylphenidate.

Grilly and Loveland (2001) reviewed the effects of different doses of amphetamine on rat behaviour. Performance-enhancing effects were seen only after relatively low doses (0.1–0.4 mg/kg). Higher doses (0.4–1.0 mg/kg) increased rates of responding but not necessarily accuracy. After very high doses (>3.0 mg/kg) performance was completely disrupted by the emergence of persistent stereotyped behaviour.

Studies of amphetamine in human subjects were stimulated by the use of the drug by the military on both sides of the Atlantic in the Second World War to counteract effects of fatigue and sleep deprivation during long missions. The numerous earlier studies have been reviewed by Weiss and Laties (1962) and Grinspoon and Hedblom (1975). The general conclusion of these studies was that low doses of amphetamine improved performance in tasks that required a long period of sustained attention, and could restore performance that had deteriorated because of fatigue or sleep deprivation.

However, the performance-enhancing effects of the drug were most apparent in situations where subjects were required to undertake simple, prolonged, repetitive, and often boring tasks. The aspect of cognition which is most likely to be affected by the drug is 'vigilance'. Koelega (1993) reviewed the literature on the effects of amphetamine on vigilance in a variety of studies on human subjects. Amphetamine was found to improve performance in eight of the 12 studies reviewed, usually by reducing the decrement in performance that otherwise occurred with time. Support for this view is also given by various studies of the performance-enhancing effects of D-amphetamine in sleep-deprived subjects (Kornetsky *et al.* 1959). Magill *et al.* (2003) found that the performance of healthy young men on a variety of cognitive and motor tasks was reduced after overnight sleep deprivation. Administration of D-amphetamine (20 mg) or phentermine (37.5 mg) partly reversed these decrements. Newhouse *et al.* (1989), in an even more severe test, deprived their subjects of sleep for a total of 60 hours. This led to marked decrements in cognitive performance in a variety of tests, but D-amphetamine (20 mg) was able to reverse these deficits almost completely.

Amphetamines dramatically decrease sleepiness, increase latency to fall asleep, and increase latency to onset of rapid eye movement (dreaming) sleep (Rechtschaffen and Maron 1964; Oswald 1968). These effects underlie the use of amphetamines by those who need to stay awake and remain vigilant for long periods of time (e.g. truck drivers, military personnel) (see Chapter 4).

There have been few human laboratory studies of the effects of D-methamphetamine on cognitive function. Johnson *et al.* (2000) reported that administration of D-methamphetamine (0.21 and 0.42 mg/kg) to healthy normal subjects improved attention, accuracy of reasoning ability, and performance on various computerized cognitive function tests. However, at these relatively high doses methamphetamine also caused adverse effects on cardiovascular function (increased heart rate and blood pressure).

There are considerable individual differences in the effects of amphetamines on human cognitive performance. Some of the underlying neurobiological reasons for these differences have become apparent in recent years. It is generally believed that the effects of amphetamine on attention and cognition are mediated principally by the drug-induced release of dopamine in the prefrontal cortex. Mattay *et al.* (2000) have suggested that dopamine impacts on prefrontal cortex function in accordance with an inverted-U dose–response curve; the response is optimum within a narrow range of released dopamine, with too little or too much having deleterious effects. Using brain imaging techniques and psychological testing with complex tests of working memory they found that D-amphetamine improved brain function and memory only in those subjects who had relatively low working memory capacity at baseline, whereas it worsened performance in subjects with a high working memory capacity at baseline. Mattay *et al.* (2003) suggested that some of these individual differences in drug response may be genetically determined. They studied different variants of the enzyme catechol-O-methyltransferase (COMT) in people with different levels of responsiveness to the memory-enhancing actions of amphetamine. COMT degrades dopamine to the inactive metabolite 3-methoxytyramine. From previous animal studies COMT was known to have an important role in the inactivation of dopamine in the brain, particularly in the prefrontal cortex where levels of the dopamine reuptake transporter are relatively low. Mice that are genetically engineered to eliminate expression of the COMT enzyme have increased levels of dopamine in the prefrontal cortex but not in the striatum, where dopamine reuptake sites are abundant (Gogos *et al.* 1998). In humans, COMT exists in two genetically determined variants which differ by only one amino acid at position 158 in the protein. The val[158] form of the enzyme is fully active, but the met[158] variant (in which methionine substitutes for valine) is very much less active. Mattay *et al.* (2003) found that individuals with two copies of the met[158] form of the enzyme (one copy inherited from each parent) tended to have above-average prefrontal cortex function and working memory capacity and they also failed to show any positive response to amphetamine; if anything, the drug worsened their performance. In contrast, individuals with two copies of the val[158] form of COMT had lower initial performance levels but showed significant improvements in response to amphetamine. These results suggest that people with two copies of the met[158] version of COMT have an impaired ability to dispose of dopamine in the brain and thus are normally exposed to higher baseline levels of dopamine; further drug-induced rises in dopamine are deleterious rather than beneficial. These are important genetic differences since approximately a quarter of the population have two copies of the met[15] gene and thus may be expected to react unfavourably to amphetamines.

Individual differences in subjective responses to amphetamines have also been attributed in part to genetically determined differences in the dopamine transporter protein, a key mediator of the drug's actions (see section 2.5).

Despite these individual differences, there is little evidence that amphetamine can truly be regarded as a 'smart' drug. A variety of studies have shown no significant effects of the drug on various cognitive tests or measures of intelligence, although it may improve attention and vigilance (Kornetsky 1958; Grinspoon and Hedblom 1975). For example, in one study 94 college students received Benzedrine or placebo in a double-blind manner and then were set a number of tests. While the drug caused a small increase in reading speed, this was offset by significantly poorer performance in tests of mental arithmetic or in devising analogies. Grinspoon and Hedblom (1975) described this subjective report from a student who had taken Benzedrine prior to an examination:

> . . . My mind worked very rapidly and seemed to be able to consider one idea after another with great speed. My hands were sweating. I felt impatient at the slowness of my writing, but I was writing at top speed. I wasn't confused. I felt 'hot' intellectually, as though I were at my very keenest. My mind was racing, yet I felt that I had complete control of the sequence of thought and was capable of ordinary thinking. It seemed that my memory was clearer and working better than ever. About ten-thirty I reached the climax of stimulation. I felt happy, powerful, quick—every faculty sharpened. I took a deep breath and resisted an impulse to laugh and tell my neighbor how good I felt.

Unfortunately, despite this drug-inspired confidence, the student's actual examination performance was mediocre. This may be an example of the postulated 'inverted U' dose–response curve for amphetamine-induced effects on cognitive performance (Laties and Weiss 1981). As the dose of stimulant increases, behaviour becomes progressively more constricted and repetitive, resulting in both cognitive and behavioural perseveration.

2.8. Stereotyped behaviour in human amphetamine users

The Swedish psychiatrist Rylander suggested the term 'punding' to describe this form of amphetamine-induced stereotyped behaviour in Swedish abusers of the dieting drug phenmetrazine. Rylander (1971) defined punding as 'an organized goal-directed but nevertheless meaningless activity' and as 'an automatic behaviour with something of the compulsive factor, which is typical for obsessive–compulsive states'. Amphetamine users, particularly those taking high doses regularly, may indulge in a variety of repetitive behaviours, including repeated car washing, home cleaning, elaborate sorting of small objects, or the endless dismantling and attempted reassembly of radios, clocks, or other mechanical devices. Ellinwood (1969) described some examples of amphetamine-induced punding.

> Watches, doorknobs, television sets, radios and phonographs, tape recorders, typewriters and children's toys were among the common items of curiosity and analysis. Some were valueless, such as old television sets from the junk yard. Many were quite expensive; one man dismantled a $1200 hi-fi set. Another sorted, filed and put on display repainted electronic parts, both new and worthless ones. This same man polished and painted everything around. He tiled his apartment, including the walls, in Armstrong pebble tiling, then painted the individual pebbles red, yellow, gold, and black . . .

Amphetamine users place great emphasis on the pleasurable nature of punding and may continue these activities for extended periods of time, and they are not easily distracted. In animals, high doses of amphetamine also induce repetitive so-called 'stereotyped behaviour' (see section 2.3). Punding is an irrational behaviour and may perhaps presage the more severe forms of psychosis that can also be induced by amphetamines (see Chapter 6).

2.9. Effects on sexual function

This is a complex topic. The effects of amphetamines are as variable as those of alcohol, and depend on dosage, personality, previous sexual experience, degree of normality of pre-drug sexual adjustment, and setting. Some amphetamine users report a decreased interest in sexual relations or even impotence. They may find the drug itself more rewarding than sex; many experienced users describe the methamphetamine high as resembling an intense orgasm. Similar brain mechanisms are involved in both the natural and the drug-induced pleasure.

However, it is also clear that many amphetamine users experience a definite increase in libidinal drive (Angrist and Sudilovsky 1978; Independent Drug Monitoring Unit 2004) which may be accompanied by delayed ejaculation or female orgasm. Promiscuity, compulsive masturbation, and prolonged intercourse with few orgasms may result—perhaps a form of the drug-induced stereotyped behaviour described in section 2.6. Kall (1992) reported the results of a study of intravenous amphetamine users in Sweden. A majority of those who had experience of sexual activity while using amphetamine reported that they became more sexually excited when on the drug and had prolonged intercourse and intensified orgasms. An American methamphetamine user describes his experience as follows.

> Then there was the sex drive. Before ever trying meth, I had a normal, healthy sex drive. When I tried meth, my sex drive skyrocketed to the point where I was so horny, if a girl even massaged my shoulders I would start panting and trying my absolute hardest to get her to have sex with me. Sex on meth is fucking amazing and other-worldly; sensuality, response, drive, stamina and duration are all increased by a thousand-fold. When I stopped taking meth, sex didn't appeal to me anymore. Without crank, sex just seemed like a chore . . . (Erowid Experience Vaults, http://www.erowid.org/experiences/exp.php?ID=36053)

People with abnormal sexual adjustment prior to drug use seem particularly prone to a higher intensification of sexual behaviour after using amphetamine. This may include sexual fantasies, promiscuity, prostitution, sadomasochistic behaviour, exhibitionism, paedophilia, and penile mutilation.

Methamphetamine use appears to be particularly attractive to gay and bisexual men. The drug-induced release of inhibitions, delayed ejaculation, and heightened sexual pleasure are motivating factors (McNall and Ramafedi 1999). Semple *et al.* (2002) found that in the USA methamphetamine use by gay men was associated with high rates of anal sex, low rates of condom use, multiple sex partners, sexual marathons and anonymous sex. Use of the drug is associated with particular environments where sexual contact among gay men is promoted, such as sex clubs and large 'circuit' parties. Unfortunately, the tendency for drug-induced unprotected sex means that methamphetamine use in the gay community may exacerbate the already serious HIV–AIDS epidemic in this group (Halkitis *et al.* 2001; Sanello 2005).

Animal studies have yielded conflicting and confusing evidence on the effects of amphetamines on sexual behaviour (Independent Drug Monitoring Unit 2004). Some studies showed increased sexual activity, whereas others showed reduced activity. There is some evidence that the effects of amphetamine in female animals may vary over the oestrus cycle, with enhanced sensitivity in the pre-ovulatory period and reduced sensitivity in the post-ovulatory period (Diaz-Veliz *et al.* 1994). In monkeys, sexual behaviour was stimulated in both males and females (Bellarosa *et al.* 1980).

In summary, a large number of human studies find an association between chronic or heavy amphetamine use and increased sexual activity, often of a high risk nature. Consequently, amphetamine use confers an increased risk of HIV infection. However, none of these studies has resolved the issue of whether amphetamine use causes such behaviour, or whether high-risk sexual activity and amphetamine use are both symptoms of an underlying risk-taking or sensation-seeking personality.

In contrast, some heavy amphetamine users experience a reduced desire for sexual contacts and may even become impotent. Nevertheless, the evidence suggests that enhanced sexual energy, stamina, and intensification of sexual enjoyment are factors that are commonly sought by amphetamine users.

2.10. Appetite suppression

In one of the first systematic studies of the effects of amphetamine on normal human subjects Bahnsen *et al.* (1938) noted that their drug-treated subjects commonly reported a reduction in appetite. Shortly after this the first positive results from clinical trials of amphetamine in the treatment of obesity were published (Lesses and Myerson 1938), and amphetamines soon became widely adopted as appetite suppressants. A more detailed review of the remarkable story of the rise and fall of amphetamines as anti-obesity agents is given in Chapter 3.

Use of amphetamines can lead to significant weight loss, at least initially. However, the appetite-suppressant effect tends to wane after some weeks of treatment and users may compensate by increasing the dose, thus exposing them to a heightened risk of becoming dependent on the drug (Grinspoon and

Hedblom 1975). Furthermore, as with other anti-obesity drugs, when amphetamine use is terminated body weight tends to revert to the starting baseline (see Chapter 3).

Exactly how amphetamines cause appetite suppression is still not clear. Complex nerve circuits in the hypothalamus, a small region lying at the base of the frontal part of the brain, control the balance between hunger and satiety which ultimately determines body weight. There has been a significant increase in scientific understanding of these mechanisms in recent years, and it is now known that a series of hormones generated in the stomach, gut, and fat tissues act on appetite-stimulating and appetite-suppressing regions of the hypothalamus to maintain normal body weight (Neary *et al.* 2004).

There is a large literature on the neurochemical mechanisms that underlie amphetamine-induced appetite suppression in animals (Hoebel 1977). The principal site of action seems to be within the hypothalamus, and the ability of amphetamines to induce the release of dopamine, norepinephrine, and serotonin may all contribute. The amphetamine derivative fenfluramine, which for a while was a highly successful anti-obesity drug, appears to act principally through its ability to cause a release of serotonin.

One of the effects of amphetamine administration in animals is to cause an increase in the synthesis of a brain chemical known as 'CART peptide'. CART stands for 'cocaine and amphetamine regulated transcript', and it was discovered by looking to see which gene products were switched on in response to cocaine or amphetamine. CART is a particularly potent appetite suppressant and it is present in the relevant parts of the hypothalamic circuits involved in appetite control. It is also found in regions of the brain associated with pleasure and reward mechanisms, which are dopamine-rich areas. It is likely that the increased synthesis of CART, turned on indirectly by amphetamine via dopamine release, plays an important part in the anorectic actions of the amphetamines (Thim *et al.* 1998; Larsen *et al.* 2002).

CHAPTER 3

Medical uses of amphetamines

Estimated legal production of amphetamine tablets in the United States in
1970 = 10 000 000 000

(Grinspoon and Hedblom 1975)

3.1. Introduction

Amphetamine was first introduced into medicine as the 'Benzedrine inhaler' in
1932, followed soon after by pill forms of the drug. As with many new medicines,
amphetamine was at first embraced enthusiastically by the medical profession
as a valuable and completely safe treatment for many ailments and it rapidly
became enormously popular. It was only later that the potential hazards associated with amphetamine use became apparent. In a review of the literature,
Reifenstein and Davidoff (1939) were able to quote 115 papers published
between 1935 and 1938 on various potential therapeutic applications for
Benzedrine. By 1946, the US physician W. R. Bett was able to describe 39 'clinical uses' (Bett 1946). These included epilepsy, Parkinson's disease, schizophrenia, alcoholism, barbiturate intoxication, anaesthetic overdose, morphine and
codeine addictions, tobacco smoking, behavioural problems in children, enur-
esis, migraine, heart block, multiple sclerosis, myasthenia gravis, myotonia
(muscular rigidity), infantile cerebral palsy, urticaria, dysmenorrhoea, colic,
irradiation sickness, and hypotension (low blood pressure). Bett was not alone
among US physicians, who rated amphetamine almost as highly as aspirin. This
may now seem naive, but it is worth remembering that the range of medicines
available to doctors in the 1940s was very limited; effective treatments for most
of the conditions listed were not available. However, in practice the genuine
medical uses of amphetamine proved to be far more limited and few of the
original indications remain current today. We have come to recognize that
amphetamines are both potentially addictive and quite toxic. In this chapter we
will review the medical uses which gained most acceptance, even though most
of these are no longer current.

3.2. Amphetamine inhalers as decongestants

The first medical use of amphetamine made use of the fact that it acts as a 'sympathomimetic' amine, promoting the release of norepinephrine from sympathetic nerve terminals in the periphery (Chapter 2). Scientists at the drug company Smith Kline and French (SKF) found that inhaled amphetamine had a beneficial effect in constricting blood vessels in the nasal cavity and dilating the bronchial tubes in the lung, and thus could be used to treat the symptoms of the common cold, hay fever, or asthma. The company licensed the patents for amphetamine from the British chemist Gordon Alles and launched the Benzedrine inhaler in 1932. This was a simple device containing quite a large amount (about 350 mg) of Benzedrine (DL-amphetamine) as the free base in oil form impregnated in cotton strips inside a simple inhaler device (Fig. 3.1).

Because amphetamine oil is quite volatile, even at room temperature, sniffing the inhaler gave the patient a small dose of Benzedrine and some degree of relief from nasal congestion and/or wheeziness in the lungs. The device could continue to deliver Benzedrine for several weeks. There is no doubt that this was effective, and the Benzedrine inhaler was hugely successful; it remained on the market in one form or another for more than 25 years. Although SKF held the patents on the Benzedrine inhaler, it was widely copied by other companies using other compounds from the amphetamine family. Burroughs Wellcome marketed an inhaler containing methamphetamine, Wyeth Laboratories had the 'Wyamine inhaler' containing the amphetamine analogue mephentermine (N-methyl analogue of phentermine; see Fig. 2.2), and there were several others. However, it was soon discovered that the Benzedrine inhaler could be a source of amphetamine for those more attracted by the euphoriant effects than by treatment of the common cold (Grinspoon and Hedblom 1975). The 350 mg of Benzedrine free

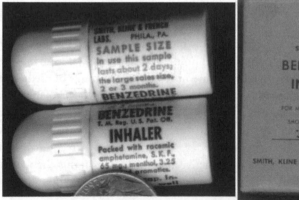
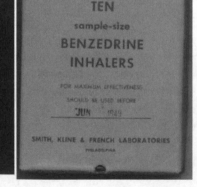

Figure 3.1 Benzedrine inhaler.

base that was present in each inhaler was equivalent to 560 mg of amphetamine sulphate, enough for many large doses when the inhaler was broken open and the contents ingested or injected (see Chapter 5). Increasing evidence of abuse led SKF to decide voluntarily to stop marketing the Benzedrine inhaler in 1949. They replaced it with the Benzedrex inhaler which contained proplyhexedrinc, a sympathomimetic amine which, although still effective as a decongestant, is devoid of central stimulant properties and abuse potential. Other companies were less scrupulous, and amphetamine- and methamphetamine-containing inhalers continued to be freely available until they were finally banned by the Food and Drug Administration (FDA) in the USA in 1959. Even then several companies continued to market inhalers containing other amphetamine-like drugs. One mid-western company even continued to sell the 'Valo inhaler', containing 150 mg of methamphetamine after the 1959 ban, and the Wyaminc inhaler containing the amphetamine analogue mephentermine continued to be sold over the counter until 1971 and was also misused (Angrist et al. 1970). Although effective in their medical uses, amphetamine inhalers introduced hundreds of thousands of people on both sides of the Atlantic to amphetamine abuse.

Even today, over-the-counter inhalers containing amphetamine-like drugs are still available as decongestants, although the compounds now used are ones that act solely on the norepinephrine system in the peripheral sympathetic nervous system and are devoid of psychostimulant properties or abuse potential. A little known fact is that the popular 'Vick inhaler' contains 50 mg of methamphetamine (described on the label by the synonym deoxyephedrine) in free base oil form; however, it is not the psychoactive D-isomer of the drug but L-methamphetamine, which has no psychostimulant properties but retains some sympathomimetic activity. Innocent users of the Vick inhaler to treat the symptoms of the common cold can get into trouble with the law if subjected to a drugs test, as this will indicate the presence of methamphetamine unless the test is sufficiently sophisticated to tell the difference between the L- and D-isomers of the drug!

3.3. Narcolepsy

Narcolepsy is a strange medical condition marked by an uncontrollable desire for sleep and sudden attacks of sleep during the waking day. Onset of the illness usually occurs between the ages of 10 and 20 and it remains as a lifetime disorder. It is estimated that 50 000–100 000 people suffer from this condition in the USA. Obviously the symptoms are not only inconvenient but can be dangerous to those whose jobs require them to stay awake and alert (e.g. drivers, miners, those in control of complex machinery). Narcolepsy was one of the first medical conditions to gain official approval for amphetamine use. The American Medical Association (1937) recommended this as one of the conditions for which Benzedrine was effective, citing positive clinical trial data from Prinzmetal and Bloomberg (1935). This was followed by many other positive reports. D-Amphetamine or methylphenidate taken twice a day is usually very effective. Until recently these remained widely used treatments for narcolepsy, but a new medicine, modafinil (trade name Provigil), seems likely to replace the amphetamines. Modafinil is not an amphetamine, but it is able to prolong wakefulness in narcoleptics and even in normal people without an unpleasant hangover effect and with no abuse potential. The mechanism of action remains unknown, but the advantages of having a non-scheduled and apparently safe medicine are obvious (Ferraro et al. 1997; Banerjee et al. 2004).

3.4. Depression

The American Medical Association (1937) also recommended Benzedrine as 'useful' in the treatment of 'certain depressive psychopathic conditions' when used 'under the strict supervision of a physician'. They spoke of the drug's ability to promote 'a sense of increased energy or capacity for work, or a feeling of exhilaration'. However, the clinical data underlying this recommendation were far less convincing (Guttmann 1936; Myerson 1936). Guttmann (1936), rediscovering what Alles (1928) had discovered several years earlier in experiments on himself, commented on the mood-elevating effects of Benzedrine in a study of the relation between the effects of the drug on blood pressure and mental phenomena. Guttmann subsequently published reports on the beneficial euphoriant effects of Benzedrine in depressed patients, although in one study (Guttmann and Sargant 1937) he reported that while the drug was effective in mildly depressed patients, it could make those with severe depression worse by provoking or intensifying anxiety. This paper ended with the prophetic statement:

> The possibility of addiction needs to be guarded against and the case of a person who has been purchasing Benzedrine at chemist's shops without medical supervision has already come to our notice, although none of our patients have so far shown a tendency to addiction . . . At present, however, Benzedrine may be purchased at any chemist's shop without prescription and this seems inadvisable with a drug all the properties of which have yet to be fully investigated . . . . It is hoped that this drug will not be discredited by misuse. (Guttmann and Sargant 1937)

Benzedrine was freely available as an over-the-counter medicine until 1939, when in the USA it became available on prescription only. Despite the weakness of the evidence, Benzedrine and other amphetamine products became widely used for a time in the treatment of depression (Fig. 3.2). In his enthusiastic review of the place of Benzedrine in medicine, Bett (1946) enthused that:

> A large number of clinical observations both from general practitioners and from specialists testify to [amphetamine's] immediate, and often dramatic, value in

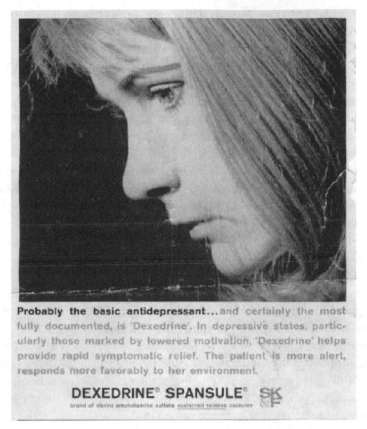

Probably the basic antidepressant... and certainly the most fully documented, is 'Dexedrine'. In depressive states, particularly those marked by lowered motivation, 'Dexedrine' helps provide rapid symptomatic relief. The patient is more alert, responds more favorably to her environment.

DEXEDRINE® SPANSULE® SK
brand of dextro amphetamine sulfate sustained release capsules

Figure 3.2 Early advertisement for Dexedrine as an antidepressant (1940s). (www.amphetamines.com/dexedrine.jpg)

breaking the stranglehold of depression, restoring 'energy feeling', and renewing optimism, self-assurance, increased initiative, appetite for work and zest for living.

It must be remembered that during the 1940s there were none of the highly effective antidepressant drugs that are available today. Physicians of that era also had little concept of how to conduct controlled clinical trials. In particular, little or no allowance was made for the fact that depression often shows spontaneous improvements. Nowadays any clinical trial of a new antidepressant drug would automatically include a comparison of groups of depressed patients receiving the active drug with another group receiving only dummy (placebo) pills. Neither doctor nor patient must know whether an individual subject is receiving drug or placebo (double blind). Even so, clinical trials of antidepressants are notoriously difficult to conduct because there is nearly always a significant improvement in the placebo group as well as in the drug-treated group.

The clinical experience with amphetamines in the treatment of depression soon made it clear that many patients reacted unfavourably, and that there were cardiovascular and abuse hazards. Drug companies attempted to counter the increasing awareness of the dangers of amphetamine by introducing new amphetamine-like drugs. One of these was methylphenidate (Ritalin), later to become famous in the treatment of behavioural disturbances in children (see section 3.5). It was claimed that methylphenidate elevated the mood of depressed patients without causing insomnia or anxiety (Nathensohn 1956; Landman *et al.* 1958). However, subsequent clinical trials failed to confirm this; most properly controlled trials found methylphenidate to be no more effective than placebo (Robin and Weisberg 1958; Thal 1969).

Another strategy used to counter the psychostimulant effects of amphetamine, particularly in causing insomnia and anxiety, was to combine amphetamine with a sedative barbiturate (Gottlieb 1949). These combinations began to be marketed under a variety of brand names (e.g. Dexamyl, Amber), but in reality the strategy was not effective. In a controlled clinical trial the British physician David Wheatley compared a combination of 5 mg D-amphetamine and 65 mg amobarbital with the individual components and placebo in groups of depressed patients (Wheatley 1969). There was no difference between D-amphetamine or the combination and placebo, and Wheatley concluded that amphetamines, whether alone or combined with barbiturates, had no place in the treatment of depression. Nevertheless, drug companies, seeing a large new market, continued to produce the combination products until they were eventually displaced by a new generation of safer and more effective antidepressants. For a while, particularly in the UK during the 1950s and 1960s, the combination drugs became very popular and were subject to abuse and black market dealing.

3.5. Amphetamines as anti-obesity agents

For more than 50 years, in the post-war period of prosperity, obesity has been seen as an increasingly important public health problem in many Western countries, none more so than the USA. People have been only too willing to believe that medicines could help them lose weight, and drug companies have been happy to oblige by providing diet pills. This became a major profitable market for the companies, and amphetamines and amphetamine-like drugs played a key role. There have been many unforeseen consequences, and some catastrophic tragedies, as this story developed.

Amphetamine has a well-recognized ability to suppress appetite, perhaps acting through its effect in increasing the synthesis of the CART peptide in the hypothalamic feeding centres of the brain (see Chapter 2). After the first clinical reports of the use of Benzedrine as an anti-obesity agent (Lesses and Myerson 1938), it was approved for this use by the FDA in 1939, followed a few years later by approval of methamphetamine also for this indication. The FDA stated: 'The sympathomimetic amines have been found of value, when administered under the supervision of a physician, as an adjunct to the dietary management of obesity'.

The amphetamines rapidly became extremely popular diet pills. By 1948 more than 90 per cent of US physicians were using them to treat obesity, and some two-thirds of patients seeking treatment for obesity were receiving them (Grinspoon and Hedblom 1975). The initial clinical studies were followed by a series of further trials and reports, many poorly designed and inadequately controlled. Physicians were slow to recognize the adverse side effects inherent in amphetamine use. For example, Finch (1947) advocated the use of D-amphetamine to control weight gain in pregnant women. He stated: 'Dexedrine is a nontoxic safe drug which may safely be used in obstetric patients to aid them in preventing excessive gain of weight'.

The patients who lost most weight appeared to be those who ate least, and so the main effect of the amphetamines seemed to be to reduce appetite rather than to increase activity levels or basal metabolic rate. The rationale for using amphetamines was that it might make it easier to adhere to a dietary regime that demanded a lower food consumption than the dieter would normal desire. Amphetamines were generally combined with dietary restrictions and for the first few weeks of treatment they were often very effective. Adlersberg and Mayer (1949) studied a total of 299 obese patients and found that those following dietary restriction plus amphetamine (5 or 10 mg twice daily) lost more weight than those on diet alone. However, they also found that the most impressive weight losses for diet alone or diet plus amphetamine occurred in the first 1–2 months of the trial. After several months the effectiveness of amphetamine wore off and higher doses had to be given to maintain weight loss; eventually there was little difference between the diet alone and diet plus amphetamine groups. Similar findings were reported by Gelvin and McGavack (1949). They studied 27 obese patients who were permitted to eat as much as they wanted. They were treated with 15 mg D-amphetamine per day, increased to 30 mg per day. After 8 weeks 47 per cent maintained a weight loss of 1 lb per week, but after 12 weeks only 23 per cent continued to lose that much. Twenty weeks after the start of the trial only one patient was still losing weight. The development of tolerance to the appetite-suppressant effects of amphetamines and the need to increase the dose, thus risking the development of addiction, meant that in practice these drugs were of only limited usefulness.

In addition, although the psychostimulant properties of amphetamine were initially disregarded, some patients suffered severely from these effects. Grinspoon and Hedblom (1975) gave the following personal account of the experience of a 25-year-old obese woman treated with amphetamine.

> I was convinced, because I was not told otherwise, that these magic little pills
> would solve my weight problem, which was substantial, amounting to an excess of
> 50 pounds. I would eventually be thin. I filled the prescription and the next morning
> took the first pill . . . . The day passed uneventfully and so did the evening (fat girls

don't go out), and then I got ready to go to bed. And couldn't. What's the sense in going to bed if you can't go to sleep, and this eluded me? I was so 'high' that my mind was running circles around itself. My thought patterns resembled Joyce's stream of consciousness technique; I could not concentrate on any thought for more than a matter of seconds and then my mind would dart to something else, seemingly unrelated. To say the least I was disconcerted because I had no control over my thoughts . . . . The next day was little better but eventually, as I recall, my tolerance built up quickly, and I did not have nighttime 'highs' after a couple of weeks. My weight problem was much more persistent. I found that Dexedrine did depress my appetite as long as my will power was in high gear; when I slipped I became a compulsive snacker, eating literally anything and everything I could get my hands on. When will power took the reins again, I would manage to drop a few pounds.

Weeks and months passed, and I remember thinking that the pills were no longer doing their job. I experienced a craving to take more than one pill a day, but never quite had the courage to do so. I also found myself becoming jittery and jumpy. Minor things would unnerve me and I tended to want to be alone more and more; I became progressively unhappy and would burst into tears over the most trivial things. I remember a period of strange, weird dreams, where I was thin, lovely, and the centre of attraction. Then I would wake up to fat reality.

After six months, I began to question the validity of continuing; I wasn't losing weight, and I was miserable in the bargain . . . I became alternatively moody, euphoric, depressed. I would snap at people for no reason at all, and was generally 'bitchy' to those around me.

In April I decided to stop taking 'the magic diet pills'

(After recovering from amphetamine withdrawal symptoms, she later went on to join Weight Watchers and lost 51 lb.)

Of course, not all those treated with amphetamines had such harrowing experiences, and many patients found that the pills did help them to lose weight, although much of this would often be regained after treatment stopped.

The recognition that many patients could not tolerate the high doses of amphetamine needed for sustained weight loss because of their psychostimulant effects led to the development of new medicines in which amphetamine was combined with a sedative barbiturate to counteract the stimulant effects, although there was little evidence that these medicines were any more effective or safe (Shapiro and Michaile 1956; Necheles and Sorter 1957). Eventually, the FDA recognized the limited usefulness of the amphetamine barbiturate combinations, stating that they differed '. . . neither in efficacy or in the incidence of adverse side effects from anorectic drugs alone' (FDA Bulletin 1972).

The pharmaceutical industry also introduced a range of new once-daily amphetamine formulations and a family of new amphetamine-like drugs, claiming each time that they had retained the desired effects on weight loss while removing any liability to over-stimulation or addiction. In the period

Table 3.1 Affinities of some amphetamine-like appetite suppressant drugs for human brain monoamine transporters

Compound	K_i (nM)		
	Norepinephrine	Serotonin	Dopamine
Phentermine	244	13 900	1580
DL-Phenmetrazine	153	>10 000	607
DL-Fenfluramine	1987	269	23 700
D-Fenfluramine	1290	150	22 000
DL-Norfenfluramine	242	480	4305
Chlorphentermine	451	338	3940
Aminorex	55	1244	216

K_i, nanomolar concentration needed to occupy half of the monoamine transporter sites.
Data from Rothman and Baumann 2003.

between 1956 and 1960 alone these included the novel drugs phendimetrazine, phentermine, benzphetamine, phenmetrazine and diethylpropion. These drugs all share the same basic amphetamine-like chemical skeleton (Fig. 2.2) and all act as monoamine-releasing agents in brain, with much the same effects and side effects as the parent amphetamines, although this conclusion was strenuously denied by the manufacturers. The affinities of some of these compounds for the monoamine transporters in brain are summarized in Table 3.1.

Modell (1960) reviewed the newer agents and concluded:

> It seems unlikely that any minor structural change in this group which continues the same theme will separate the effect on appetite from the other effects of the central stimulant action that may be clinically undesirable. Yet it is precisely this which is inferred from many claims made for these drugs, namely the recurrent claims for reduced incidence of insomnia, anxiety and nervousness, with potent anorectic effect.

The quality of the scientific data supporting claims for these new drugs was often very poor, even though the results were published in reputable scientific and medical journals. The standards of rigour for clinical trials were not very high 50 years ago. The paper by Freed and Hays (1959) is an example of the genre. They reported on a new formulation of the dieting drug phentermine. In the preparation, which was called Ionamin, phentermine was linked to an ion exchange resin, giving a formulation that released the drug gradually in the gastrointestinal tract for absorption into blood. The paper does not indicate how the subjects were selected or how obese they were at the start of the trial. No control (placebo) or D-amphetamine comparator groups were included, and the data presented are sparse, although the conclusion was that subjects treated with 30 mg phentermine daily lost an average of 7 lb over the 1-month period of the trial. The authors minimized the importance of adverse side effects, describing the insomnia that patients often experienced as 'somewhat different from that occurring during amphetamine therapy'; their patients 'reported a wakefulness which was not unpleasant, compared to the nervous overexhilaration which prevented sleep following amphetamine treatment'. The authors concluded that Ionamin was '. . . chemically and pharmacologically different from amphetamine'.

Modell and Reader (1970), in their review of anorectic agents, gave a more accurate verdict on phentermine: 'All systemic effects, therefore, stem from an amphetamine-like action. There is no good evidence that this is in any way a superior member of the group'.

In Europe the amphetamines and amphetamine-like drugs also proved popular as anti-obesity agents. In addition to the amphetamine-like drugs introduced in the USA, there were some that were used in Europe but never registered in the USA. A combination of caffeine and ephedrine known as the 'Elsinore pill', which was invented in Denmark, was popular for a while (Malchow-Møller et al. 1981) and is still available.

Another tragic example was the compound aminorex (Fishman 1999). Aminorex had the traditional dopamine/norepinephrine-releasing properties of other amphetamines, but in addition it had other pharmacology. Notably, it impaired the normally rapid removal of serotonin from the blood as it passes through the lungs and it also acted to constrict the arteries carrying blood to the lungs (Weir et al. 1996). None of this was known when the drug was first marketed, but these features may explain why aminorex was associated with an outbreak of the serious lung disease primary pulmonary hypertension (PPH) in Europe during the 1960s. PPH is a distressing and often progressive condition in which the pulmonary blood vessels carrying blood to the lungs are constricted, leading to impaired oxygenation and fluid accumulation in the lungs. Patients literally drown in their own fluids, gasping for breath. In many cases PPH is irreversible and leads to death. Fortunately, PPH is a rare disease with an incidence of 1–2 per million in the normal population. Although manufactured by an American company, McNeil Laboratories, aminorex was never approved for use in the USA. However, it became a popular anti-obesity agent in some European countries, capturing 80 per cent of the market for such medicines in Switzerland and also selling well in Austria and Germany. In late 1967 an astute Swiss physician, Gurtner, noted a dramatic and unexplained 20-fold increase in the numbers of patients with PPH coming for treatment at the University Medical Clinic, Bern. He noted that most of the new patients were obese and most had been taking aminorex. Ingestion of more than eight packs of aminorex tablets over a period of months was associated with a 10 per cent risk of developing PPH. The patients with drug-induced PPH had the classical pathology of spontaneous PPH cases, but their disease often progressed rapidly and although some showed reversal when the drug was stopped, many became progressively worse and died. Gurtner and his colleagues were cautious in interpreting their findings as proof that aminorex was the cause of the new spate of PPH cases, but nevertheless the Swiss authorities withdrew the drug from sale in 1968, and similar action followed later in Austria and Germany, the two other European countries in which the drug had found favour. In the USA, McNeil Laboratories withdrew their application for approval of the drug by the FDA and discontinued further development, but by then the damage had been done. In total, some 600 patients in Switzerland, Austria, and Germany may have developed PPH as a result of taking aminorex between 1967 and 1969. The numbers of new cases dropped dramatically after the withdrawal of the drug. The aminorex 'epidemic' should have acted as a warning for the future that the effects of new appetite suppressants on the lungs should be carefully monitored, but this did not happen, with further tragic consequences. This may in part be due to the fact that the Swiss findings were largely published in German-language journals and the data took some time to reach an English-speaking readership (Follath *et al.* 1971; Gurtner 1985). Even then a cause-and-effect relationship between aminorex and PPH was not always accepted; it was argued that less than 2 per cent of patients treated with the drug developed PPH, and animals treated with high doses of aminorex had not exhibited any signs of pulmonary changes (*Lancet* 1971). The aminorex episode was soon forgotten.

Despite the doubtful efficacy and safety of amphetamines in the treatment of obesity their use grew to remarkable proportions as figures for the USA show (Colman 2004):

• 1958: 3.5 billion tablets
• 1967: 8 billion tablets
• 1967: 23 million prescriptions (80 per cent female).

A large proportion of these prescription drugs were being diverted to other non-medical uses. However, important changes were on the way in USA. In 1962 the Kefauver–Harris amendments to US drug approval laws meant that in future the FDA would require that prescription drugs be shown to be clinically effective as well as safe to use in patients (previously only safety had to be demonstrated). The FDA established a number of panels of experts to undertake a retrospective review of the efficacy of amphetamines as anti-obesity agents. By 1970, their conclusion was that amphetamine-like drugs were at best 'possibly effective' and there were several criticisms of the data available in the literature. Studies were of short duration, there was no available evidence that the drugs altered the natural history of obesity, there was some evidence that the anorectic effects may have been strongly influenced by the suggestibility of the patient, and there were concerns about the adequacy of the controls in some of the clinical studies (Colman 2004).

The FDA set up further advisory groups to formulate a formal policy on the approval of anorectic drugs. In 1971 guidelines were issued requiring that a statistically significant difference be demonstrated between drug-treated and placebo groups, and that clinical trials be at least of 12 weeks duration. European regulatory agencies soon followed suit with similar recommendations.

The FDA went on establish the Amphetamine–Anorectic Drug Project, which undertook a meta-analysis of clinical data submitted to FDA for all amphetamine and amphetamine-like compounds. There were 200 clinical studies involving 10 000 patients. The conclusions were that patients treated with active medication lost 'some fraction of a pound a week more than those on placebo'. However, the data did not suggest that one drug was superior to another. The FDA stated:

> . . . all anorectic drugs including amphetamines and methamphetamines have a limited usefulness in the treatment of obesity, and because of their significant potential for dependence and abuse should be used with extreme care. (Colman 2004)

Nevertheless, as a result of this analysis, in 1973 the FDA stopped short of an outright ban and declared that amphetamine and amphetamine-like drugs were to some extent effective for the treatment of obesity, although concerns about abuse led the FDA to impose a short-term (a few weeks) limit on all amphetamine and amphetamine-like drugs for this use. These warnings did have some effect. A review of 450 US physicians in 1973 (Lasagna 1973) showed that 73 per cent rated the abuse potential of amphetamines as 'very high'. Nevertheless, about two-thirds continued to prescribe them for obesity.

The FDA continued to be concerned about the use of amphetamines as anti-obesity agents and in 1979 called for removal of the obesity indication for D-amphetamine and methamphetamine, arguing that there was no evidence that these drugs were more effective for treating obesity than the other supposedly safer amphetamine-like drugs. In reality none of the amphetamines or their congeners resulted in much more than a 3 kg loss of weight, and this was very likely to relapse once treatment was stopped.

FDA requirements for approval of new anorectic agents have become progressively more stringent. Guidelines issued in 1996 require that clinical trial data show that the mean weight loss in the drug group is at least 5 per cent greater than the mean weight loss in the placebo group; in addition, the proportion of patients who lose at least 5 per cent of baseline weight must be greater in the drug group than in the placebo group. Clinical trials should include at least 1500 patients studied for 1 year under placebo-controlled conditions and 200–500 patients for an additional year of open-label study.

Despite these new hurdles, new drugs continued to be approved in Europe and the USA. The most notable additions were fenfluramine and its optical isomer D-fenfluramine (dexfenfluramine). If aminorex had proved to be a health hazard, fenfluramine was to become a disaster of epic proportions. Its use would result in serious heart or lung disease in nearly half a million people in the USA, and an untold number in Europe, and it would trigger the largest mass tort lawsuit ever seen in American legal history. The story is well told in the book *Dispensing with the Truth* (Mundy 2001).

Although fenfluramine shares some of the characteristic chemical features of other amphetamines it differs radically in its pharmacology from the compounds discussed previously. The drug appears to have its principal action on serotonin mechanisms in the brain, rather than dopamine. It is taken up by the serotonin transporter and can displace serotonin (see Chapter 2), and it was initially thought that increased drug-induced levels of serotonin in the hypothalamic appetite control centres in the brain might explain its anorectic action (Curzon and Gibson 1999). However, experiments in animals showed that blockade of the serotonin transporter by the selective inhibitor fluoxetine (Prozac®) blocked the ability of fenfluramine to release serotonin in rat brain but did not prevent its appetite-suppressant action. Similarly, treatment of animals with the serotonin synthesis inhibitor PCPA (p-chlorophenyl-amphetamine) blocked the serotonin-releasing action without preventing appetite suppression (Curzon and Gibson 1999). It seems likely that the ability of fenfluramine to act directly on some subtypes of serotonin receptor in brain may be the key to its anorectic actions (Curzon *et al.* 1997). Fenfluramine is recognized by a number of serotonin-receptor subtypes in brain (NIMH Psychoactive Drug Screening Program, http://kidb.cwru.edu); in addition, it can interact directly with norepinephrine receptors in the α-subtype family and has weak dopamine-blocking activity. The latter may explain why fenfluramine, unlike traditional amphetamines, is sedative rather than stimulant.

Fenfluramine was approved for use in Europe and the USA in the 1970s and was marketed as a mixture of D- and L-isomers under the trade name Pondimin in the USA. However, the unwanted sedative actions limited the popularity of fenfluramine as an anti-obesity medicine. People who had to work or look after children were reluctant to take it for more than few weeks because of the drug-induced drowsiness.

Sales of DL-fenfluramine (Pondimin) received an unexpected boost in the 1990s as a result of a momentous new discovery when Mike Weintraub, a research scientist at the University of Rochester with an interest in the pharmacological treatment of obesity, hit upon a novel idea. Since the problem with fenfluramine was too much sedation and the problem with old-fashioned amphetamine-like drugs was the opposite, why not combine the two of them?

Thus was born the famous, and later infamous, Fen–Phen cocktail in which fen-fluramine was combined with the older amphetamine-like drug phentermine (Fig. 2.2). Weintraub did not undertake any animal experiments, but launched a lengthy clinical trial of this new drug combination in 121 obese people, chart-ing their weight over a 4-year period. The studies were completed in the 1980s, but the results were not published in full until 1992 (Weintraub 1992). The findings were dramatic, with the subjects showing sustained weight loss over this period. Perhaps more importantly, the study appeared to show that it was possible to undertake long-term treatment with anti-obesity medicines safely and with minimal side effects.

A. H. Robins, the company that controlled sales of DL-fenfluramine (Pondimin) in the USA under license from Wyeth, was acquired by Wyeth, who saw a potential for boosting sales of the flagging fenfluramine product. Although the companies decided not to explore the difficult path of gaining FDA approval for a combination product, they helped to promote the 'off-label' use of the Fen–Phen combination (Mundy 2001). It is alleged that some of the financial support for Weintraub's research came from Wyeth–Robins, and after his results were published they helped to disseminate them. Reprints of his pub-lication landed in doctors' offices around the country and on the desks of health writers at major newspapers and magazines. The story received prominent cov-erage in women's magazines, and in the *Reader's Digest*. The idea of a safe new medicine that caused substantial weight loss and could be used over long peri-ods of time caught the public imagination and the Fen–Phen frenzy took off in the USA. Neither Wyeth nor the companies selling phentermine could under-take overt advertising for Fen–Phen as it was not an FDA approved medicine; nevertheless, their 'soft' promotion campaigns proved highly successful, as the sales figures showed (Table 3.2).

Weintraub's clinical data on the Fen–Phen combination were later given added support by results from animal studies showing that the two drugs had synergistic rather than merely additive interactions. The drug combination had a greater effect in suppressing appetite and boosting brain serotonin levels than either alone, suggesting that it was possible to use lower doses of each drug and yet maintain adequate appetite control with minimal side effects (Wellman and Maher 1999).

Table 3.2 Number of prescriptions for phentermine and fenfluramine in the USA

	1992	1996
Phentermine	2 000 000	11 000 000
Fenfluramine	69 000	7 000 000

Data from Colman (2004).

Another way of improving the profile of fenfluramine emerged from research in France and the USA which showed that in animals and humans the D-isomer of fenfluramine (dexfenfluramine) retained the appetite-suppressant properties but was much less sedative. In France, Jacques Servier, the founder of Servier Laboratories, saw dexfenfluramine as a way of expanding his company's sales of anti-obesity medicines after the original patents on DL-fenfluramine expired. He launched dexfenfluramine in Europe in 1987 under the trade name Isomeride, and initial sales were very successful. In the USA, Dick and Judith Wurtman, a husband-and-wife team of scientists at Massachusetts Institute of Technology, also showed the advantages of dexfenfluramine as a less sedative anorectic agent in animal experiments and filed a patent covering this use in the USA in 1980. In their research the Wurtmans had long promoted the notion that serotonin played a key role in the brain as a satiety signal controlling appetite for carbohydrates. Wurtman *et al.* (1987) claimed that dexfenfluramine had a selective effect in suppressing the intake of foods with high carbohydrate content rather than protein, and suggested that the drug would reduce the frequency of 'snacking' in obese patients prone to consuming high-carbohydrate foods. Clinical trials with dexfenfluramine showed long-term results (6–12 months) no better than those seen with traditional amphetamine-like drugs, with maximum weight losses of 2–3 kg more in the drug-treated groups than in those seen in placebo-treated groups, but the drug seemed to be well tolerated (Silverstone 1992). Dick Wurtman went on to found a commercial company, Interneuron, in 1988 to develop dexfenfluramine as an anti-obesity medicine for the US market. He formed an alliance with a large company, Wyeth, in order to develop and market the drug, a task far beyond the resources of Interneuron. At first things went well, but relations between Interneuron and Wyeth grew more complex as Wyeth saw the Fen–Phen combination emerge as a means of giving new life to the old product Pondimin, which they also owned. Nevertheless, Wyeth invested heavily in clinical trials and other development costs for dexfenfluramine, and prepared the extensive documentation needed for FDA approval.

However, the fairy story of a safe diet pill would eventually come to an abrupt end for both Fen–Phen and dexfenfluramine (Redux). While the USA was indulging in the Fen–Phen craze and the FDA was beginning to review dexfenfluramine for approval, serious worries were emerging in Europe about the safety of fenfluramine. It had long been known that some patients taking fenfluramine developed PPH as a rare adverse side effect, but on both sides of the Atlantic the risk had been considered so small that it was outweighed by the benefits of treating obesity. However, in the late 1980s hospitals in France began reporting many new cases of PPH in younger women taking the newly launched dexfenfluramine (the Fen–Phen combination was never used in

Europe). The French government commissioned Lucien Abenhaim, a prominent epidemiologist, to undertake a detailed review of the possible links between the diet drugs and PPH. The International Primary Pulmonary Hypertension Study (IPPHS) drew experts from across the world, including the USA, and after 2 years they produced their report, initially presented in draft form to the French government and to the companies involved (Servier, Interneuron, and Wyeth), and later published in final form in the *New England Journal of Medicine* (Abenhaim *et al.* 1996). The findings were damning. PPH affects only 1–2 people per million in the general population, but among patients taking fenflu-ramine or dexfenfluramine the risk was increased more than 10-fold. Furthermore, the risk increased with duration of drug treatment, rising much higher with longer use (3 months or more). French and European health officials were said to have wanted to withdraw the drugs from the market altogether, but apparently fearing the wrath of Jacques Servier, who had power-ful political allies (Mundy 2001), they announced plans merely to place severe restrictions on the use of fenfluramine and dexfenfluramine, making them available only to morbidly obese patients, and then only for a limited time. Sales of both drugs dropped precipitately. This should have prevented dexfenflu-ramine (Redux) from ever being approved in the USA. As Abenhaim said: 'We assumed that after the news about the European health authorities' decision, naturally the FDA would never approve Redux'. But he was wrong. In one of the most inexplicable episodes in its history the FDA, normally regarded as a hard-nosed evidence-based organization, did go on to approve Redux, despite warnings from many of the experts involved in an advisory capacity. However, the approval process was tortuous.

In addition to the risk of drug-induced PPH, Wyeth had to argue against strong opposition from some members of the neuroscience community in the USA, who worried about the possible neurotoxic actions of dexfenfluramine. It had been known for some time that fenfluramine caused a long-lasting depletion of serotonin from the brain in laboratory animals, including rats, mice, guinea pigs, and monkeys, and some studies had suggested that this was accompanied by actual damage to the distal terminals of serotonin-containing nerves (Molliver and Molliver 1990; Sotelo 1991). As in the similar case of ecstasy-induced dam-age to the serotonin system in brain (see Chapter 8) the husband-and-wife team of Una McCann and George Ricaurte in Baltimore contributed data and warned against the possible dangers of brain damage caused by Redux (McCann *et al.* 1997a). Dick Wurtman at Interneuron believed that the findings from the ani-mal experiments had been over-dramatized, and accused Ricaurte of 'running a cottage industry showing that everything under the sun is neurotoxic'.

The FDA Advisory Committee for Redux, a group of scientific and medical experts convened to advise the FDA, met in September 1995 to consider the approval of the drug. Committee members heard directly from Lucien Abenhaim about the IPPHS findings. Wyeth downplayed his findings and argued that the risk of PPH, although real, was minor and likely to affect only small number of patients. They cited the statistic of 300 000 deaths from obesity annually in the USA as a counter-argument, claiming that obesity was a public health crisis in the USA that could be helped by Redux, although it was never clear what the origin of this statistic was. Warnings about possible human neurotoxicity were given to the Committee by two prominent US neuroscientists, Lewis Seiden and Mark Molliver. Wyeth again downplayed these findings, arguing that there was no evidence for human neurotoxicity. The Committee discussed the possibility of approving Redux under the condition that the risks of PPH and neurotoxicity would be rigorously monitored after marketing the drug had started, in a so called 'Phase 4' study. Finally, the Advisory Committee voted against approval by 5–3. The meeting ended in some disarray and some members departed prematurely; almost incomprehensibly the Chairman said that he would have to reschedule another meeting to vote again. The second meeting was held in November 1995, and this time the neuroscientists Seiden and Molliver were not present as they were attending the annual meeting of the Society for Neuroscience in California. Despite continuing concerns about PPH and neurotoxicity, the vote this time went in favour of Redux, but by the smallest of margins (6–5).

In May 1996 Redux was launched on the US market with a $52 million public relations and advertising campaign from Wyeth. Media interest was high, and sales of both Redux and the older drug Pondimin took off. Wyeth stood to make a profit of $180 million on the two drugs that year, with some 6 million patients using the drugs in the USA. Redux had one of the fastest sales build-ups of any new prescription medicine ever, and was rapidly heading towards the magic $1 billion annual sales within the first 2 years. This was despite the fact that the final report of the IPPHS published only a few months after the Redux launch showed even higher risk figures than those estimated in the earlier draft report, suggesting that patients who took the drugs for more than 3 months ran a 23-fold increased risk of developing PPH. However, the impact of this publication was blunted by an accompanying Editorial in the *New England Journal of Medicine* (Manson and Faich 1996) which denigrated the IPPHS report and concluded:

> Obesity is an escalating problem in the United States, and the condition is notoriously difficult to treat. Because the associated health hazards are considerable, medications are needed that produce and maintain weight loss safely and effectively. Dexfenfluramine is an important new drug in the clinician's arsenal, but it is not free of risk. Although physicians and patients need to be informed, the possible risk of pulmonary hypertension associated with

dexfenfluramine is small and appears to be outweighed by benefits when the drug is used appropriately.

It was only later that the journal learned that the authors of this Editorial were hardly unbiased commentators; both had acted as consultants to Wyeth and had given evidence in favour of Redux at the FDA hearings!

However, if the risks of drug-induced PPH and possible brain damage were bad, what was to come next was far worse. In the mid-West town of Fargo, North Dakota, an observant medical technician, Pam Ruff, who ran echocar-diogram equipment (a technique which used ultrasound to image the beating human heart) at the local hospital, began to notice an unusual incidence of heart valve defects in young women, many of whom had been taking the Fen–Phen combination. She alerted the hospital cardiologists and one of these, Jack Cary, eventually became seriously concerned. He contacted colleagues at the Mayo Clinic, Rochester, Minnesota, who had also seen instances of similar heart valve defects in patients taking the diet drugs. They pooled their data on the first 24 cases and published a brief report in the *New England Journal of Medicine* in August 1997 (Connolly *et al.* 1997). In view of the serious implications of their findings, the journal allowed the authors to make the data public before publication and placed an advance copy of the paper on the journal website, both highly unusual moves. If the findings from North Dakota and the Mayo Clinic were extrapolated, they implied that as many as a quarter or a third of patients taking Fen–Phen for 3 months or more were at risk of heart valve damage—a potential public health disaster. The high incidence of heart valve defects implied by the initial data dwarfed the risk of drug-induced PPH which, although real, was far smaller. On 8 July 1997 the Mayo Clinic held a nationally televised press conference to publicize the findings, and the story led the network television news that night across the USA. Thousands of diet drug patients panicked and stopped taking their medicines immediately. Sales of Pondimin, Redux, and phentermine rapidly began to drop. Meanwhile the doctors from Fargo and the Mayo Clinic had provided their data to both Wyeth and the FDA as they were accumulated, although neither recipient appeared to have taken them very seriously to begin with. Later lawsuits would even accuse Wyeth of deliberately covering up the initial evidence of this serious drug-induced side effect. In Fargo the local hospital was sufficiently concerned that they issued a ban on any further use of the Fen–Phen combination or the new drug Redux. Another immediate consequence was the damage done to the alliance between Interneuron and Wyeth. Incredibly, Wyeth had not kept Interneuron informed of the developing heart valve problem, so that when executives from both companies were invited to attend an emergency meeting at the FDA to review the problem, Interneuron did not know what hit them.

As Mundy (2001) put it, two of the leading scientists in the Fen–Phen and Redux stories, Dick Wurtman and Mike Weintraub,

> ... found themselves sucked into the vortex of corporate pharmaceuticals, where academics were disposable accessories. Scholars who made cracks about barracuda fights in think tanks suddenly found themselves in real shark tanks when they got involved with drug companies.

The initial report of heart valve problems was rapidly followed by the description of 28 additional cases (Graham and Green 1997). Of the initial 52 patients, 11 were sufficiently ill to require heart surgery. Heart valve defects were seen in patients treated with fenfluramine (Pondimin) or dexfenfluramine (Redux) alone, but they were more common in people taking the Fen–Phen combination (Seghatol and Rigolin 2002). It appears that fenfluramine and dexfenfluramine or their metabolites acted directly on serotonin receptors of the 5-HT-2B subtype on the heart valves to cause cell proliferation and scar tissue formation (Fitzgerald et al. 2000), or they caused sufficient elevation of blood levels of serotonin to achieve the same result. In addition, fenfluramine and dexfenfluramine, like aminorex, contracted pulmonary arteries, increasing the risk of PPH (Weir et al. 1996; Fishman 1999). Furthermore, animal experiments indicated that the Fen–Phen combination acted synergistically to enhance neurotoxicity (McCann et al. 1997a, 1998a; MacLean 1999; Wellman and Maher 1999).

Wyeth fought a desperate rearguard action to keep Redux and Pondimin on the market, at first denying the validity of the heart valve findings and refusing to accept that any causal relationship had been established. In July 1997 they were forced by FDA to include a 'black box' in the label inserted into every package of drug, warning patients of valvular heart disease or PPH, but still denying any cause-and-effect relationship. However, by August 1997 the FDA had received reports on 58 cases of heart valve defects in patients taking Fen–Phen or Redux and it was clearly only a matter of time before the drugs would have to be voluntarily or forcibly withdrawn. Wyeth and Interneuron finally agreed to a 'voluntary' recall of both drugs in September 1997.

What followed was the largest civil legal action ever seen in the USA, as patients who had possibly experienced heart valve damage joined a mass legal action against Wyeth and Interneuron. More than 300 000 people, mostly women, were represented in this action which was eventually successful, largely because juries were convinced that Wyeth had deliberately withheld or delayed crucial early warning data on the heart valve problem from the FDA. By November 2004 the company had paid out or reserved $16 billion in damages for fenfluramine or dexfenfluramine claims. Another 62 000 patients decided not to join the mass settlement, but to sue Wyeth and its parent company

American Home Products directly. Some of these cases still await trial, but many proved highly successful. By February 2005 Wyeth had increased their estimate of the total cost of Fen–Phen litigation to a staggering $22.1 billion.

The outcome of this dreadful episode in America was in sharp contrast to that in Europe where fenfluramine and dexfenfluramine were also withdrawn. Although European patients died as a result of drug-induced PPH and some also suffered heart valve problems, no-one sued and no payments were granted by juries. It is a sharp reflection of the cultural/medical differences that exist across the Atlantic that fenfluramine had been on the market in many European countries for some 20 years without reports of serious adverse effects, apart from rare instances of drug-induced PPH. Dexfenfluramine was approved in France in 1985 and subsequently in 65 other countries. By 1995 sales corresponded to 41 million patient-months (Curzon and Gibson 1999), but although reports of an increased incidence of drug-induced PPH led to the IPPHS study, there were few reports of heart valve defects. However, in the US experience such defects were often sufficiently minor as to be asymptomatic and only detectable by use of ultrasound heart scanning technology. A Belgian cardiologist, Mariane Ewalenko, had noticed six patients taking fenfluramine or dexfenfluramine who developed valvulopathies, and she reported this to the parent company Servier in 1992, but no further action was taken (Mundy 2001). After the initial furore had subsided, a more careful analysis of the US data suggested that the original estimates of as many as a third of patients developing heart valve defects may have been exaggerated; in some of the initial studies the investigators were not blinded to patient versus control groups and the estimates may have failed to take proper account of the fact that obese patients who are not treated with diet drugs have quite a high spontaneous incidence of heart valve abnormalities (up to 5 per cent) (Loke *et al.* 2002). The numerous US studies that sought to establish the true incidence of diet-drug-induced valvulopathies gave estimates as high as 31 per cent in some cases, but as low as 5 per cent in others (Seghatol and Rigolin 2002). The lawyers preferred to believe the higher figures, although the numbers of patients joining the lawsuits compared with the estimated six million US patients exposed to fenfluramine and dexfenfluramine suggest that an incidence of heart valve defect of 5–10 per cent may be the correct figure.

Given the appalling history of diet pills as relatively ineffective anti-obesity agents with a poor safety record, one might think that their day had come and gone. However, this is far from the case. In 2005 a variety of amphetamine-like medicines were still available in the USA as prescription drugs. These include benzphetamine, diethylpropion, phentermine (including the sustained-release resin Ionamin), phendimetrazine, and phenylpropanolamine (nor-pseudoephedrine). All of these are nowadays more or less freely available at various on-line pharmacies, not requiring a visit to the doctor's office. In 2000, the European Union Committee on Proprietary Medical Products recommended the withdrawal of all amphetamine-like appetite suppressants on the grounds of an 'unacceptable risk/benefit ratio'. The drugs involved were phentermine, diethylpropion, amfepramone, clobenzorex, fenproporex, mefenorex, phenyl-propanolamine (nor-pseudoephedrine), and phendimetrazine. However, this decision was challenged in the European courts by the manufacturers and by physicians (Kinnell 2003). The European Union eventually lost its case after an appeal to the European Court of Justice and the decision to withdraw the drugs had to be annulled (SCRIP, 30 July 2003).

The public appetite for a quick fix to obesity does not seem to have abated. Following the demise of fenfluramine, the new compound sibutramine, which acts as a mixed inhibitor of monoamine transporters for norepinephrine, dopamine, and serotonin, has been approved in the USA and Europe for weight loss (Arterburn et al. 2004). There have also been important advances in under-standing the complex brain mechanisms involved in appetite control and regulation of body mass, with an increasing emphasis on neuropeptides and circulating hormones (Neary et al. 2004). Pharmaceutical companies continue to view obesity as an ever-increasing area of unmet medical need and a poten-tially lucrative market for new diet pill products. They are investing millions of dollars in research in this area in the hope of achieving the ultimate goal of a safe and effective means of controlling appetite and obesity.

3.6. Amphetamines for children: treatment of attention deficit hyperactivity disorder

While other medical uses of amphetamines have been in decline in recent years, one area has seen dramatic growth—the treatment of children with ADHD. The two principal products, Ritalin (methylphenidate) and Adderall (mixed amphet-amine salts), have sales in excess of $2 billion annually, and the market is grow-ing at an annual rate of around 20 per cent (www.shire.com). It may seem paradoxical that drugs considered at high risk of abuse by adults should prove acceptable as medicines for children aged as young as 3 years! However, ADHD and its treatment by psychostimulant drugs has generated great scientific and social interest in recent years. PubMed, the US National Library of Medicine database of publications in the scientific literature, lists nearly 10 000 published articles on this subject, and a search using Google yielded 447 000 items!

3.6.1. What is ADHD?
Attention deficit hyperactivity disorder (ADHD) is a condition that becomes apparent in some children in the preschool and early school years. It is hard for

these children to control their behaviour and/or pay attention. It is estimated that 3–5 per cent of children have ADHD, or approximately 2 million children in the USA. This means that in a classroom of 25–30 children, it is likely that at least one will have ADHD. The term ADHD supersedes terms such as 'minimal mental dysfunction', 'minimal brain dysfunction', or 'hyperkinetic disorder' used in the earlier literature. An adult form of ADHD is also increasingly recognized. The impact of ADHD on society is enormous in terms of the stress it causes to families, adverse academic and vocational outcomes, and negative effects on self-esteem.

This remarkable story started at the turn of the twentieth century when a behavioural syndrome that resembles what we now refer to as ADHD was first described in children. The British physician Sir George Still gave a series of lectures to the Royal College of Physicians in England in which he described a group of impulsive children with significant behavioural problems that he believed were caused by a genetic dysfunction and organic brain disorder, and not by poor child rearing—children who today would easily be recognized as having ADHD (Still 1902). In the language of the time, Still described these children as suffering from 'an abnormal defect of moral control', which he defined as '. . . the control of action in conformity with the idea of the good of all'. Still gave an example of a girl who was 'wantonly mischievous' and who would throw cups, saucers, and knives at her mother, or scream and kick if disciplined.

Many studies have compared normal children with those with ADHD in an attempt to define the precise nature of the neuropsychological differences that characterize this condition. Denney and Rapport (2001) reviewed 98 such studies published between 1980 and 1999. Among those differences that were 'highly reliable' between normal and ADHD groups were tests that involved sustained attention or the ability to inhibit behaviour (impulsivity). Sustained attention tests, for example, commonly involve identifying a letter or combination of letters from a continuous list presented over a period of several minutes. Impairments were also reliably seen in tests of memory for lists of digits or pairings of words and colours. Less reliable differences were seen in more complex cognitive tasks involving planning or visual/motor control, and in general there were few differences in tests of verbal fluency or motor performance.

Nowadays there is an international agreement on the diagnosis of ADHD (American Psychiatric Association 2000). A good description of the characteristic features of the disorder is given in the publication *Attention Deficit Hyperactivity Disorder* issued by the US National Institute of Mental Health in 2003 (available online at: nimh.nih.gov/publicat/adhd.cfm#adhd3)

According to the most recent version of the *Diagnostic and Statistical Manual of Mental Disorders* (DSM-IV-TR) (American Psychiatric Association 2000), there are three patterns of behavior that indicate ADHD. Children with ADHD may show several signs of being consistently inattentive. They may have a pattern of being hyperactive and impulsive far more than others of their age. Or they may show all three types of behavior. This means that there are three subtypes of ADHD recognized by professionals. These are the **predominantly hyperactive-impulsive type** (that does not show significant inattention); the **predominantly inattentive type** (that does not show significant hyperactive-impulsive behavior) sometimes called ADD—an outdated term for this entire disorder; and the **combined type** (that displays both inattentive and hyperactive-impulsive symptoms).

Hyperactivity-Impulsivity

Hyperactive children always seem to be 'on the go' or constantly in motion. They dash around touching or playing with whatever is in sight, or talk incessantly. Sitting still at dinner or during a school lesson or story can be a difficult task. They squirm and fidget in their seats or roam around the room. Or they may wiggle their feet, touch everything, or noisily tap their pencil. Hyperactive teenagers or adults may feel internally restless. They often report needing to stay busy and may try to do several things at once.

Impulsive children seem unable to curb their immediate reactions or think before they act. They will often blurt out inappropriate comments, display their emotions without restraint, and act without regard for the later consequences of their conduct. Their impulsivity may make it hard for them to wait for things they want or to take their turn in games. They may grab a toy from another child or hit when they're upset. Even as teenagers or adults, they may impulsively choose to do things that have an immediate but small payoff rather than engage in activities that may take more effort yet provide much greater but delayed rewards.

Some signs of **hyperactivity-impulsivity** are:

Feeling restless, often fidgeting with hands or feet, or squirming while seated

Running, climbing, or leaving a seat in situations where sitting or quiet behavior is expected

Blurting out answers before hearing the whole question

Having difficulty waiting in line or taking turns.

Inattention

Children who are inattentive have a hard time keeping their minds on any one thing and may get bored with a task after only a few minutes. If they are doing something they really enjoy, they have no trouble paying attention. But focusing deliberate, conscious attention to organizing and completing a task or learning something new is difficult.

Homework is particularly hard for these children. They will forget to write down an assignment, or leave it at school. They will forget to bring a book home, or bring the wrong one. The homework, if finally finished, is full of errors and erasures. Homework is often accompanied by frustration for both parent and child.

The DSM-IV-TR gives these signs of **inattention:**

Often becoming easily distracted by irrelevant sights and sounds

Often failing to pay attention to details and making careless mistakes

Rarely following instructions carefully and completely losing or forgetting things like toys, or pencils, books, and tools needed for a task

Often skipping from one uncompleted activity to another.

Children diagnosed with the Predominantly Inattentive Type of ADHD are seldom impulsive or hyperactive, yet they have significant problems paying attention. They appear to be daydreaming, 'spacey', easily confused, slow moving, and lethargic. They may have difficulty processing information as quickly and accurately as other children. When the teacher gives oral or even written instructions, this child has a hard time understanding what he or she is supposed to do and makes frequent mistakes. Yet the child may sit quietly, unobtrusively, and even appear to be working but not fully attending to or understanding the task and the instructions.

These children don't show significant problems with impulsivity and overactivity in the classroom, on the school ground, or at home. They may get along better with other children than the more impulsive and hyperactive types of ADHD, and they may not have the same sorts of social problems so common with the combined type of ADHD. So often their problems with inattention are overlooked. But they need help just as much as children with other types of ADHD, who cause more obvious problems in the classroom.

Is It Really ADHD?

Not everyone who is overly hyperactive, inattentive, or impulsive has ADHD. Since most people sometimes blurt out things they didn't mean to say, or jump from one task to another, or become disorganized and forgetful, how can specialists tell if the problem is ADHD?

Because everyone shows some of these behaviors at times, the diagnosis requires that such behavior be demonstrated to a degree that is inappropriate for the person's age. The diagnostic guidelines also contain specific requirements for determining when the symptoms indicate ADHD. The behaviors must appear early in life, before age 7, and continue for at least 6 months. Above all, the behaviors must create a real handicap in at least two areas of a person's life such as in the schoolroom, on the playground, at home, in the community, or in social settings. So someone who shows some symptoms but whose schoolwork or friendships are not impaired by these behaviors would not be diagnosed with ADHD. Nor would a child who seems overly active on the playground but functions well elsewhere receive an ADHD diagnosis.

To assess whether a child has ADHD, specialists consider several critical questions: Are these behaviors excessive, long-term, and pervasive? That is, do they occur more often than in other children the same age? Are they a continuous problem, not just a response to a temporary situation? Do the behaviors occur in several settings or only in one specific place like the playground or in the schoolroom? The person's pattern of behavior is compared against a set of criteria and characteristics of the disorder as listed in the DSM-IV-TR.

Despite these seemingly clear diagnostic criteria, the borderline between ADHD and what might be termed 'boisterous mischief' remains hard to define. There are transatlantic differences in rates of diagnosis; until recently European doctors seemed more reluctant that those in the USA to diagnose ADHD. As a consequence US children currently account for 85 per cent of the world sales of amphetamines and amphetamine-like drugs for the treatment of ADHD. However, the transatlantic differences may be diminishing. The UK Department of Health reported that, in 2004, 5 per cent of British schoolchildren met the diagnostic criteria for ADHD, and prescriptions for Ritalin and other amphetamines had risen to almost 350 000 from 270 000 in 2003.

The reality of life with a child suffering from ADHD is vividly depicted in the following excerpt from an article in *Time* magazine:

> Dusty Nash, an angelic-looking blond child of seven, awoke at 5 one recent morning in his Chicago home and proceeded to throw a fit. He wailed. He kicked. Every muscle in his 50-lb body flew in furious motion. Finally, after about 30 minutes, Dusty pulled himself together sufficiently to head downstairs for breakfast. While his mother bustled about the kitchen, the hyperkinetic child pulled a box of Kix cereal from the cupboard and sat on a chair.
>
> But sitting still was not in the cards this morning. After grabbing some cereal with his hands, he began kicking the box, scattering little round corn puffs across the room. Next he turned his attention to the TV set, or rather, the table supporting it. The table was covered with a checkerboard Con-Tact paper, and Dusty began peeling it off. Then he became intrigued with the spilled cereal and started stomping it to bits. At this point his mother interceded. In a firm but calm voice she told her son to get the stand-up dust pan and broom and clean up the mess. Dusty got out the dust pan but forgot the rest of the order. Within seconds he was dismantling the plastic dust pan, piece by piece. His next project: grabbing three rolls of toilet paper from the bathroom and unraveling them around the house.
>
> It was only 7:30, and his mother Kyle Nash, who teaches a medical-school course on death and dying, was already feeling half dead from exhaustion. Dusty was to see his doctors that day at 4, and they had asked her not to give the boy the drug he usually takes to control his hyperactivity and attention problems, a condition known as attention deficit hyperactivity disorder (ADHD). It was going to be a very long day without help from Ritalin. (Claudia Wallis, *Time*, 18 July 1994)

3.6.2. The neurobiology of ADHD

Numerous studies have sought to investigate the genetic and psychosocial factors that contribute to the disorder, and to understand what abnormalities exist in the brains of patients with ADHD (Faraone and Biederman 1998). A number of family studies have shown that ADHD runs in families; parents exhibiting symptoms of adult ADHD have a 1 in 4 risk of having a child with ADHD. Studies of identical twins have shown a concordance rate of 0.8, i.e: if one twin develops ADHD the other has an 80 per cent chance of also developing the disorder. The fact that the concordance rate in identical twins is not 100 per cent suggests that although genetic factors are important, environment may also play a part. There is also some evidence that the genetic risk of ADHD is linked to familial vulnerability to depression and possibly to bipolar disorder (Faraone and Biederman 1998). More detailed genetic analysis has suggested that ADHD may be caused by several interacting genes rather than a single gene. Thus ADHD fits into the common genetic models of psychiatric illnesses, which have a complex multi-gene basis. Bobb *et al.* (2005) reviewed over 100 studies that have examined the genetics of ADHD by linkage or association, seeking to identify the genes responsible. These included three genome-wide linkage studies and association studies of 94 polymorphisms in 33 candidate genes. While no definite conclusions can yet be reached, consistent evidence for association exists for four genes in ADHD: the dopamine D_4 and D_5 receptors, and the dopamine and serotonin transporters. Others are promising but need further replication, including the dopamine D_2 and serotonin 2A receptors. It is notable that three of the four genes for which evidence of association is strongest are associated with dopamine function in the brain, suggesting the possibility that ADHD is associated with abnormalities in dopamine systems.

Many aspects of the biological and psychosocial environment have also been examined as potential risk factors for ADHD (Faraone and Biederman 1998). A number of speculative hypotheses have attempted to link dietary lead poisoning, excess sugar intake, or synthetic food additives with ADHD, but systematic studies failed to support these ideas. However, psychosocial risk factors appear to play a real and important role. Rutter's now classic studies of psychosocial risk factors for childhood mental disorders, including ADHD, led the way (Rutter *et al.* 1975). He studied the prevalence of mental disorders among children living in very different environments in the UK: the middle-class affluence of the Isle of Wight, and a deprived area of inner London. This research revealed six risk factors that correlated with childhood mental disturbances: severe marital discord, low social class, large family size, paternal criminality, maternal mental disorder, and foster placement. The aggregate of these rather than any individual factor seemed to be critical. Rutter's 'index of adversity' was later found to be positively associated with ADHD (Faraone and Biederman 1998).

Attempts to pin down specific abnormalities in brain function in ADHD have been less successful (Faraone and Biederman 1998; Solanto *et al.* 2001). There have been many studies using the most modern brain imaging techniques. Some studies using magnetic resonance imaging (MRI) have found that certain brain areas are consistently smaller in the ADHD brain; these include the right prefrontal cortex, the caudate nucleus, the globus pallidus, and a subregion of the cerebellar vermis. Imaging studies that aimed to detect functional changes in brain blood flow or glucose metabolism have yielded inconsistent results; with some showing increased activation of frontal cortex and others reduced activation in subjects undertaking a variety of mental tasks (Solanto *et al.* 2001). Again, it is interesting to note that, with the exception of the cerebellum, the brain regions implicated all receive a dopaminergic input. However, ADHD remains a poorly understood disorder in terms of the nature of the brain malfunction underlying it, or the molecular genetic basis.

3.6.3. Chemistry and pharmacology of methylphenidate (Ritalin) and Adderall

Methylphenidate

Methylphenidate (MP) (trade name Ritalin) was first synthesized in 1944 and was marketed by the Ciba-Geigy pharmaceutical company, which later became Novartis (Fig. 3.3). The compound exists in several isomeric forms; the racemic

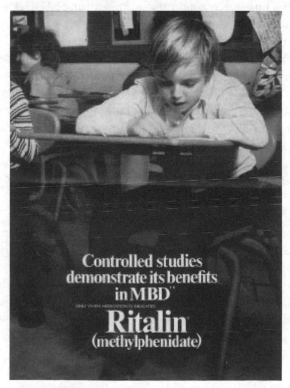

Figure 3.3 Early example of an advertisement for Ritalin for ADHD, which was formerly known as minimal brain dysfunction (MBD). (www.amphetamines.com/methylphenidate/ ritalinkid.html)

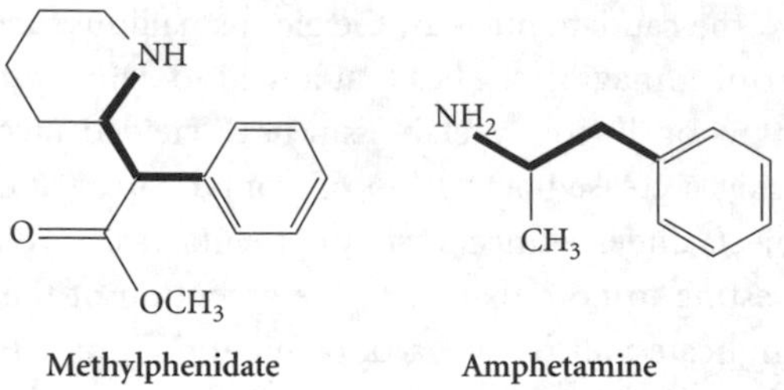

Methylphenidate   Amphetamine

Figure 3.4 Structures of methylphenidate (Ritalin) and amphetamine. Some chemical bonds are highlighted in bold to illustrate the chemical similarities between the compounds.

mixture of the D- and L-isomers of *threo*-methylphenidate which is used medically. The *erythro* forms of MP were removed in the 1950s because they caused elevated blood pressure (Swanson and Volkow 2001). MP was introduced as a medicine because, like D-amphetamine, it alleviated fatigue and stimulated mental and physical performance. It was initially recommended for the treatment of chronic fatigue, lethargy, disturbed senile behaviour, depression, and narcolepsy. Virtually all these uses have been abandoned and the use of MP is now largely confined to the treatment of ADHD, where it is the most widely used pharmaceutical (Leonard *et al.* 2004).

MP bears an obvious structural resemblance to D-amphetamine (Fig. 3.4) and it is also closely similar in its pharmacology. MP is a potent inhibitor of dopamine and norepinephrine uptake in monoamine neurons by virtue of its affinity for the catecholamine transporters (Ferris *et al.* 1972; Gatley *et al.* 1996). However, unlike D-amphetamine, MP has little affinity for the serotonin transporter, and it is less effective than D-amphetamine in displacing catecholamines from their vesicular storage sites (Kuczenski and Segal 1997). The affinities for monoamine transporters are as follows: norepinephrine transporter, 37 nM; serotonin transporter, > 10 000 nM; dopamine transporter, 345 nM (NIMH Psychoactive Drug Screening Program; available online at http://kidb.cwru.edu/). When given to rats by intravenous injection it causes a rapid and substantial increase in the rate of release of both dopamine and norepinephrine in brain, comparable to the effects of D-amphetamine (Hurd and Ungerstedt 1989; Kuczenski and Segal 1997). However, unlike D-amphetamine, MP does not cause any increase in serotonin release in rat brain (Kuczenski and Segal 1997). In rats, MP elicits behavioural changes similar to those seen after D-amphetamine, with increased locomotor activity followed by repetitive stereotyped behaviour after large doses. The behaviourally active doses corresponded to those which caused significant increases in catecholamine release in rat brain (Kuczenski and Segal 1997). In terms of both behavioural stimulation and its ability to promote catecholamine release in the brain, MP is approximately 10 times less potent than D-amphetamine.

Using brain imaging techniques, Volkow and colleagues at the Brookhaven National Laboratory (Volkow *et al.* 1999; Swanson and Volkow 2003) showed that clinical doses of orally administered MP caused more than 50 per cent blockade of the dopamine transporter sites in brain, comparable to the effect of the powerful psychostimulant drug cocaine which also acts as an inhibitor of dopamine uptake in brain. However, unlike cocaine, orally administered MP does not cause marked euphoria and is unlikely to lead to dependence. Swanson and Volkow (2003) argued that this is because the onset of the effect of MP on the dopamine transporter is slow, whereas that of cocaine is very rapid. This seems to be an example of the phenomenon discussed previously, i.e. the rate at which drugs enter the brain and bind to their targets plays a crucial part in their reinforcing and addictive properties. Grace (2001) has argued that slowly absorbed psychostimulants, such as MP, can only mimic the 'tonic' function of dopamine in the brain, which is normally activated by a constant low level of dopamine release. When dopamine neurons are activated to fire in bursts, a surge of dopamine is available at the synapse to mediate 'phasic' functions (Grace 2000). This can only be mimicked by drugs that are delivered rapidly to the brain, allowing sufficient build-up of dopamine to simulate that achieved by rapid neuronal discharge. It is argued that it is the 'phasic' mode of dopamine release that is associated with euphoria and reward. A subsequent imaging study from the same laboratory (Volkow *et al.* 2004) showed that clinical doses of MP were able to cause increased release of dopamine in human brain, but the effect was most marked when subjects were asked to undertake a challenging mental arithmetic task as opposed to passively viewing cards. This illustrates an important difference between MP and D-amphetamine. As an inhibitor of dopamine reuptake with little ability to displace the vesicle stores of dopamine, MP will enhance dopamine levels in brain most effectively only in those brain regions where dopamine is being released, such as during a difficult mental task. In this respect MP may differ qualitatively from D-amphetamine which causes dopamine release irrespective of the underlying activity state of the dopamine neurons.

MP is rapidly absorbed after oral administration, with peak drug levels in plasma within 1–3 hours. However, there is considerable degradation of the drug by liver metabolism before it enters the bloodstream, and the extent of this varies markedly between individuals (Swanson and Volkow 2001; Leonard *et al.* 2004). Consequently there is a wide range of individual variability in plasma drug concentrations for a given dose of MP. The proportion of MP actually entering the bloodstream unchanged (oral bioavailability) ranges from 11 to 53 per cent in children (Chan *et al.* 1983). The drug also has a relatively short duration of action because it is rapidly metabolized and eliminated, giving an effective duration of only about 3–4 hours. These factors mean that the optimum dose of MP varies among individuals, and when treatment is started the dose has to be gradually increased to determine this (Wolraich and Doffing 2004). The short duration of action also means that the drug needs to be taken more than once a day, creating difficulties for schools in managing drug dosing and offering opportunities for inappropriate use of drug supplies. This problem has been partly overcome by the development of slow-release formulations of MP (trade names: Concerta and Metadate) which extend the duration of action to 7–8 hours, making drug administration during the school day unnecessary (Swanson and Volkow 2001; Leonard *et al.* 2004). A further development has been the marketing of D-MP as a separate single-isomer form of the drug (trade names Focalin and Attenade) (Keating and Figgit 2002). The D-isomer appears to account for essentially all of the activity of DL-MP. Human brain imaging studies showed that L-MP penetrates the brain together with D-MP, but in animal behavioural experiments it was devoid of stimulant actions (Ding *et al.* 2004). The use of D-MP allows the dose of MP to be halved and there is a small increase in duration of action, but apart from this there seems to be no real scientific advantage in using the single isomer. Another pharmaceutical advance is the development of a skin-patch formulation for delivering MP (Methypatch) (in advanced stages of development by Shire Pharmaceuticals); this should permit an even greater extension of the duration of action of MP, with attendant advantages of convenience and minimization of risk of abuse. Another approach is the development of a prodrug form of MP chemically linked to an amino acid. The conjugate is pharmacologically inert and can only release MP when digested in the gut, thus precluding administration by any other route (www.shire.com/shirepharma).

Adderall

MP is by far the most widely used compound for the treatment of ADHD, but a second medicine Adderall®, has become popular in recent years and in 2004 accounted for nearly a quarter of the US sales of prescription medicines for ADHD. Adderall was first developed more than 20 years ago by Rexar Pharmaceuticals in the USA as Obetrol, and was marketed as an appetite suppressant. It is a complex mixture of different salt forms of amphetamine, containing D- and L-amphetamine sulphate, D- and L-amphetamine aspartate, and D-amphetamine saccharate, with a ratio of D- to L-amphetamine of 3:1. There seems little rationale for this mixture, except perhaps to distinguish Obetrol from other amphetamine products marketed at the time. Clinical trials comparing D- and L-amphetamine in treating hyperactive children have shown that L-amphetamine is effective although, as expected, less so than the pharmacologically more potent D-isomer (Arnold *et al.* 1972; Gross 1976). Adderall has a duration of action of 6–7 hours, and this has been extended further by the preparation of a slow-release formulation (Adderall-XR®) (McGough *et al.* 2003). Comparisons of Adderall with MP have shown the two drugs to be of similar efficacy, although the longer duration of action of Adderall compared with standard-release MP gives it some advantages (Arnold 2000; Faraone *et al.* 2002).

3.6.4. What are the effects of amphetamines in children and adults with ADHD?

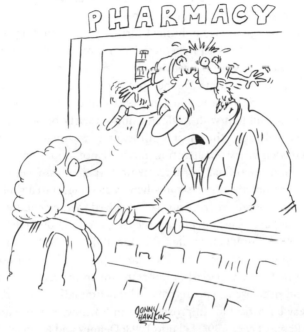

"I might suggest Ritalin."

The first evidence for beneficial effects of amphetamine in children was reported by Bradley (1937). He studied 30 children (aged 5–14years) of normal intelligence suffering from a variety of behavioural disturbances sufficiently severe to be admitted to hospital. They were treated with a daily dose of Benzedrine (DL-amphetamine) for 1 week. Several obvious changes in behaviour were observed, including subdued emotional responses and less aggressive, noisy, or domineering behaviour. However, most remarkable were changes in school behaviour.

> Possibly the most remarkable change in behaviour during the week of Benzedrine therapy occurred in the school activities of many of these patients. Fourteen children responded in a spectacular fashion. Different teachers, reporting on these patients, who varied in age and school accomplishment, agreed that a great

increase of interest in school material was noted immediately. There appeared a definite 'drive' to accomplish as much as possible during the school period, and often to spend extra time completing additional work. Speed of comprehension and accuracy of performance were increased in most cases. Insight into school improvement was generally present, though few of the children attributed it to the medication they had received earlier in the day. The improvement was noted in all school subjects. It appeared promptly the first day Benzedrine was given and disappeared on the first day it was discontinued. (Bradley 1937)

Is it any wonder that many parents with behaviourally disturbed children have given Ritalin and Adderall a warm welcome?

Bradley and Bowen (1941) published further positive findings from clinical studies in 100 children with hyperactivity and other behavioural disorders undergoing treatment with Benzedrine. Most subsequent work was done with MP rather than amphetamine. Denney and Rapport (2001) reviewed 50 different studies published between 1961 and 1991 that compared the effect of MP with placebo in children with ADHD, using a variety of neuropsychological tests. Not surprisingly, the most significant and consistent drug-induced benefits were seen in tests of attention and vigilance, impulsivity (matching to sample, reaction time), and learning/memory (paired associations, spelling). MP had little or no effect on tests involving visual/perceptual skills or perceptual/motor tasks. Some experiments have involved treating children with drugs that blocked dopamine or norepinephrine receptor function in the brain before receiving MP. The results indicated that the ability of MP to stimulate both dopamine and norepinephrine function are important, but that dopaminergic stimulation may be particularly important for improvements in attention/vigilance and decreased hyperactivity, while stimulation of norepinephrine function may be critical for improvements in learning/memory and planning functions (Rapport *et al.* 1993; Solanto 1998; Denney and Rapport 2001; Mehta *et al.* 2001). A review of the cognitive-enhancing effects of amphetamine and MP in normal volunteers also concluded that both the dopamine and the norepinephrine systems were involved (Mehta *et al.* 2001).

How can one explain the apparently paradoxical effects of psychostimulants in calming children with ADHD and improving their cognitive function? One hypothesis invokes the theory of rate dependency for CNS drug actions. Rate dependency refers to the observation that low baseline rates of response are increased by a drug, whereas higher rates are found to increase to a lesser extent or to decrease as a result of drug treatment. Thus response rate is an inverse function of baseline rate, as described in the model

$$\log(D/C) = (a-b)\log C$$

where D is the response rate on the drug, C is the baseline response rate, and a and b are constants (Dews and Winger 1977).

Many studies in a wide range of species, reviewed by Dews and Winger (1977), have documented rate-dependent effects of amphetamine on fixed-interval and fixed-ratio schedules of reinforcement. Such effects have been shown for amphetamine doses as low as 0.1 mg/kg, with doses between 0.3 and 1.0 mg/kg found to produce decreases in high base rate responding. Thus it appears that decreases in motor activity can be produced by amphetamines at doses lower than those which generate stereotypy and associated reduction in locomotor activity.

Robbins and Sahakian (1979) postulated that the decrease in spontaneous motor activity seen in children with ADHD after treatment with stimulant drugs is attributable to rate-dependent effects. Their re-analysis of raw data from several drug studies of ADHD children yielded a good fit to the rate-dependency equation. In particular, re-analysis of data from the NIMH study of drug effects on normal children, normal adults, and children with ADHD (Rapoport et al. 1980) yielded a slope of -0.65 for the plot of drug response rate as a function of base rate. Whereas both groups of children showed a decrease in activity on 0.5 mg/kg D-amphetamine, normal men, who had as a group much lower activity counts at baseline, showed a very small (but statistically significant) decrease only on the lower of the two D-amphetamine doses (0.25 and 0.5 mg/kg) they received. Furthermore, the greatest reductions in activity were found for the most active ADHD children, whereas increases in activity were found for some normal adults within the group. A subsequent study of children with ADHD by Solanto (1986) also reported a highly significant correlation of -0.94 between baseline spontaneous locomotor activity and the change in activity level following MP administration.

While these scientific insights are valuable, the approval of psychostimulant drugs as prescription medicines for the treatment of children with ADHD depended on more concrete evidence that they were effective and safe. A variety of different rating scales have been devised to assess the effects of these drugs on ADHD symptoms. Commonly used rating scales include the Conners Teachers' Scale and the Conners Parents' Scale (Conners 1969, 1998) and their revised forms (Conners et al. 1998), now backed up by large databases of information derived by applying these scales to large populations of normal and ADHD children of various ages. These and other similar rating scales use the diagnostic criteria for ADHD and ADD defined by DSM-IV (see above) to provide numerical scores. Converting the complex cluster of symptoms characteristic of ADHD, with the variations in symptoms between individuals, into numbers is of course an oversimplification, but in order to conduct clinical trials of drugs for treating ADHD it is a convenience as it permits statistical analysis of the resulting data. However, the results are always subject to the individual bias of teachers and parents. Nowadays, approval of a new medicine for ADHD will rely on positive data from a variety of outcome measures involving teachers, parents, and physicians, including some form of global clinical assessment measure of improvement. An example of an ADHD rating scale for teachers is shown in Table 3.3.

A recent development has been the increasing recognition that the symptoms of childhood ADHD often persist into adolescence and quite frequently into

Table 3.3 Teachers' ADHD rating scale

El Camino Pediatrics: ADHD Rating Scale-IV School Version

Child's Name _____

Child's Age _____ Sex: M F Grade _____ Child's Race _____

Circle the number that *best describes* this student's school behavior over the past 6 months (or since the beginning of the school year).

	Never or rarely	Sometimes	Often	Very often
1. Fails to give close attention to details or makes careless mistakes in schoolwork	0	1	2	3
2. Fidgets with hands or feet or squirms in seat	0	1	2	3
3. Has difficulty sustaining attention in tasks or play activities	0	1	2	3
4. Leaves seat in classroom or in other situations in which remaining seated is expected	0	1	2	3
5. Does not seem to listen when spoken to directly	0	1	2	3
6. Runs about or climbs excessively in situations in which it is inappropriate	0	1	2	3
7. Does not follow through on instructions and fails to finish work	0	1	2	3
8. Has difficulty playing or engaging in leisure activities quietly	0	1	2	3
9. Has difficulty organizing tasks and activities	0	1	2	3
10. Is 'on the go' or acts as if 'driven by a motor'	0	1	2	3
11. Avoids tasks (e.g. schoolwork, homework) that require sustained mental effort	0	1	2	3
12. Talks excessively	0	1	2	3
13. Loses things necessary for tasks or activities	0	1	2	3
14. Blurts out answers before questions have been completed	0	1	2	3
15. Is easily distracted	0	1	2	3
16. Has difficulty awaiting turn	0	1	2	3
17. Is forgetful in daily activities	0	1	2	3
18. Interrupts or intrudes on others	0	1	2	3

adulthood (Wender 2001; Wilens *et al.* 2002; Newton-Howes 2004). As many as a third of children with ADHD will continue to manifest similar symptoms in adulthood. However, the diagnosis of adult ADHD remains controversial, with no firmly agreed diagnostic criteria (McGough and Barkley 2004). A widely used self-diagnostic test is the Wender Utah Rating Scale (Ward *et al.* 1993; Wender 2001) which uses a retrospective diagnostic assessment by means of self-report on a 61-item checklist of childhood behaviour. There seems little doubt that adult ADHD is real, although the symptoms are not identical to those seen in children. Adult ADHD is often accompanied by poor academic achievement or work performance and may be associated with antisocial behaviour, depression, and anxiety disorders. Nevertheless, the same psychostimulant drugs used to treat ADHD in children are also effective in adults (Faraone *et al.* 2004; Spencer *et al.* 2004). Rating scales have been adapted for use in adult ADHD, including a version of Conners Adult Rating Scale, the Brown ADHD Scale, and ADHD Rating Scale IV. Adults and adolescents, unlike children, can also be asked to complete self-report assessment scales, for example the Adult ADHD Self Report Scale (Murphy and Adler 2004). MP and Adderall have been shown to be effective in treating the symptoms of adult ADHD (Faraone *et al.* 2004; Spencer *et al.* 2004) and are available as prescription medicines for this indication. No doubt pharmaceutical companies see adult ADHD as a new area of unmet medical need that will allow further expansion of the market for amphetamine-like psychostimulants. One company (Eli Lilly) posts a six-item self-report checklist on its website so that adults can diagnose themselves (http://www.adhd.com/adult/index.jsp)!

3.6.5. How safe are Ritalin and Adderall?
Both Ritalin and Adderall are remarkably safe drugs when used in the correct oral dosage regimes as recommended. However, as with any medicines there are adverse side effects, some of which are serious and others less so. Behavioural side effects sometimes occur that are reminiscent of the stereotyped repetitive patterns of behaviour seen in laboratory animals after high doses of amphetamine. These include abnormal movements, perseverative/compulsive behaviours, lip smacking, lip licking, and stereotyped behaviour (e.g. picking at fingernails/fingertips, rubbing eyes or face, head jerking, eye blinking, etc) (Leonard *et al.* 2004). Children treated with Ritalin or Adderall may suffer loss of appetite and sleep disturbances. Loss of appetite may be so severe that growth is significantly impeded, but both these side effects are usually controllable by adjusting the dose and ensuring that the first dose of the day is given after rather than before breakfast. There is no evidence for long-term growth impairment (Hechtman and Greenfield 2003).

The most serious adverse side effects are associated with sympathomimetic actions. As explained in Chapter 2, amphetamines and amphetamine-like drugs act on the peripheral sympathetic nervous system to promote norepinephrine release. This can cause an increase in heart rate and blood pressure, which in most healthy young people is of little consequence. However, there have been reports of serious adverse events associated with the cardiovascular system and even some deaths. This led to the temporary suspension of Adderall XR in Canada in 2005, and the FDA have announced plans for a review of cardiovascular problems and psychiatric adverse events associated with all drugs used to treat ADHD, including atomoxetine (SCRIP, 1 July 2005). These risks are heightened when children being treated with psychostimulants indulge in strenuous exercise or sports activities, which themselves activate the cardiovascular system.

Instances of abuse and dependence liability with Ritalin or Adderall are rare, but this is largely because they are administered orally and build up slowly in the brain, triggering 'tonic' rather than 'phasic' dopamine mechanisms (see above). There is little doubt that both methylphenidate and amphetamine can cause euphoria and have abuse potential if administered intravenously or by other fast-absorption routes (see below).

3.6.6. Social impact: the Ritalin Age

In the past 20 years the recognition of ADHD as one of the most common childhood psychiatric disorders and the dramatic increase in the use of psychostimulant drugs to treat it has had an enormous social impact. This is particularly notable in the USA where the use of drugs to treat ADHD has grown most rapidly, but it is also increasingly so in Europe. In the UK, the annual number of prescriptions for Ritalin was only 2000 in 1990, but rose to 92 000 by 1997 and to 350 000 by 2004. The UK National Institute for Clinical Excellence (NICE) issued guidelines for the use of Ritalin in ADHD in 2000 and these are due to be updated. In 2000 and 2001 NICE recommended that Ritalin be used only for the most severe cases of ADHD, sometimes termed hyperkinetic disorder. These children display all three of the key symptoms of inattentiveness, hyperactivity, and impulsiveness. It was estimated that this might include about 1 per cent of all schoolchildren, far less than the 5–10 per cent routinely treated with Ritalin or Adderall in the USA. Is the cautious UK approach the right one? Or does it deprive many children and families of an effective medicine? Has the prescribing of psychostimulants to both children and adults gone too far in the USA, creating problems of control and diversion of supplies to non-medical uses? The answer probably lies somewhere in mid-Atlantic between these two extremes.

In the USA, the first decade of widespread Ritalin use in the 1980s and 1990s was largely a period of optimism. As the numbers of children using the drug grew, ADHD awareness became an industry, a passion, and an almost messianic movement. In the USA an advocacy and support group called CHADD (Children and Adults with Attention Deficit Disorders) exploded from its foundation in 1987 to 28 000 members in 48 states by the mid-1990s Information bulletin boards and support groups for adults sprang up on CompuServe, Prodigy, and America Online. Numerous popular books were published on the subject, advocating increased awareness of ADHD and explaining its treatment with Ritalin. Notable among these were Barbara Ingersoll's now classic *Your Hyperactive Child*, published in 1988, and the best seller *Driven to Distraction: Recognizing and Coping with Attention Deficit Disorder from Childhood to Adulthood* by psychiatrists Edward Hallowell and John Ratey, published in 1994. The first sentence of their book was to become an accurate prophesy: 'Once you catch on to what this syndrome is all about, you'll see it everywhere'.

Summer camps designed to help children with ADHD were organized, videos and children's books appeared, and therapists, tutors, and workshops offered their services to the increasingly self-aware ADHD community. It is a community that continues to view itself with some pride. Popular books and lectures about ADHD often pointed out positive aspects of the condition. Adults with ADHD see themselves as creative; their impulsiveness can be viewed as spontaneity; hyperactivity gives them enormous energy and drive; even their distractibility has the virtue of making them alert to changes in the environment. Many ADHD adults gravitate into creative fields or work that provides an outlet for emotions.

However, CHADD overreached itself in 1995 when it petitioned the US Drug Enforcement Agency (DEA) to reclassify Ritalin from the tough Schedule II category (used for dangerous narcotics) to Schedule III, which would have made Ritalin more easily available. The DEA refused this request, and during the course of the hearings it emerged that CHADD had received substantial funding ($900 000) from the drug company Ciba-Geigy, which was then the sole supplier of Ritalin.

A variety of groups in North America opposed the use of Ritalin and denied the validity of the diagnosis of ADHD from the beginning. The Church of Scientology is traditionally opposed to modern psychiatry and to all psychotropic drugs. It has waged a persistent campaign, claiming that Ritalin represented a 'chemical straitjacket' and that children with ADHD were merely 'energetic and bored'. Scientologists waged their war against Ritalin and psychiatry through the Citizens Commission on Human Rights, a non-profit organization based in Los Angeles which was formed by the Church in 1969 to investigate mental health abuses. The Commission helped to promote a major legal action in which five separate class action suits were filed against Novartis (the manufacturer of Ritalin), the American Psychiatric Association (APA) and CHADD. All five of the suits alleged that APA and Novartis engaged in an illegal conspiracy to boost the sales of Ritalin and thus improve the company's bottom line. The suits charged that to achieve these increased profits for Novartis, APA and the drug company conspired to widen the diagnostic criteria of ADD and ADHD, which have appeared in the last several editions of DSM-IV, in an unnecessarily broad manner. The suits then alleged that APA and Novartis touted the efficacy of Ritalin as a treatment for the disorder. If successful, these lawsuits could have resulted in huge payments to the families of the children involved. However, in October 2001 the judge in the New Jersey suit, Charles Walsh of the Superior Court of New Jersey in Bergen County, ruled that the plaintiffs' claim was insufficiently specific. He gave them 90 days to provide additional material to bolster their charges. The plaintiffs did not follow through on the judge's order, and once the deadline had passed decided to withdraw their complaint.

Opposition to Ritalin and Adderall and the widespread diagnosis of ADHD in American children has grown more vociferous in recent years, and has been taken up as a campaign among the Conservative Right. A considerable negative impact followed the discovery that MP was as effective as cocaine in blocking the dopamine transporter in human brain (Volkow *et al.* 1999). These findings received much media attention, and MP was portrayed as being as hazardous as cocaine. However, as explained earlier, there is in fact a great difference between the subjective euphoriant effects of injected or smoked cocaine, which enters the brain rapidly and activates 'phasic' dopamine mechanisms, and the slow build-up of MP in the brain after oral administration, which triggers 'tonic' dopamine actions. If cocaine is taken in tablet form orally, it is absorbed slowly and is no longer a powerful euphoriant. However, such pharmaceutical nuances were not what those opposed Ritalin wanted to hear, and the analogy between MP and cocaine continues to be used repeatedly. Some of the phrases used by critics to describe Ritalin included 'kiddie cocaine', 'more potent than cocaine', 'cheap fix', 'discipline in pill form', 'legalized drug pushing to children', 'making drug addicts out of America's children', and, at the wilder fringes, 'ban Ritalin not guns' or the concept that this was all a feminist conspiracy to make boys more like girls! ADHD has been described as 'a creation of the psychiatric-pharmaceutical cartel', 'a hoax', or 'the perfect way to explain the inattention, incompetence, and inability of adults to control their kids'. Parents were accused of masking their own failings by 'doping up their children to calm them down'. Another concern that has often been voiced by critics of Ritalin is that exposing children to powerful psychotropic drugs will make them more likely to abuse drugs later in life. Along with the comparison of Ritalin to cocaine, this concept has become embedded in the popular media as proved. If true, it would indeed represent a serious social problem and provide a strong reason for limiting the use of Ritalin and related drugs. However, the evidence from longitudinal studies of the subsequent drug history of children treated with Ritalin has actually led to precisely the opposite conclusion. Although some earlier studies gave conflicting results, a meta-analysis of all the available data concluded that childhood use of Ritalin was protective against adult alcohol or drug misuse (Wilens *et al.* 2003). Use of a meta-analysis is an approach often used to reconcile conflicting findings. The method evaluates whether the aggregate evidence across all available studies provides evidence for statistically valid conclusions to be made. Wilens *et al.* (2003) analysed data from six published studies, involving a total of 674 children treated with Ritalin or related drugs and 360 unmedicated subjects. Overall, there was a statistically significant protective effect of medication. Children treated with psychostimulants were nearly six times less likely to use alcohol or illegal drugs in adolescence, and the protective effect persisted into adulthood, although reduced to an odds ratio of 1.5. A possible explanation for these findings could be that unmedicated children or adolescents with ADHD may be more likely to 'self-medicate' by seeking out alcohol or illegal psychotropic agents. Hechtman and Greenfield (2003), reviewing the long-term safety of psychostimulant use in children, also concluded that the evidence did not suggest an increased risk of substance abuse.

Some US politicians have been caught up in the campaign to restrict the use of psychostimulants in children. Several states have passed laws forbidding school staff other than those who are medically qualified to recommend the use of Ritalin or Adderall to parents or their pupils. At the other extreme, some schools have insisted that unruly children be treated with medicines. In the UK some schools threatened to expel badly behaved pupils unless they were treated with Ritalin (BBC News, 24 July 2003). In the USA, a couple in New York State faced child abuse charges when they tried to take their 7-year-old son off Ritalin. They feared that the drug was harming their son's appetite and sleep. However, after complaints from the school district social service a family court judge ruled that they must continue giving him the drug (*Albany Times Union*, 19 July 2000).

The widespread use of psychostimulants in schools and colleges is not without its problems. In the USA, with more than 2.5 million children being treated with these drugs, it is inevitable that there is some diversion of supplies and abuse. Some schoolchildren sell their prescription drug supply to others, and Ritalin tablets have become known as 'Vitamin R', 'R-ball', or 'Smart Drug'; at a price of $1.00–$5.00 per pill most can afford to try it. Some estimates suggest that as many as a quarter to a third of all schoolchildren will have tried illicit Ritalin at some time or another during their school careers. There are indications that organized drug dealers are also becoming involved in the marketing of illicit supplies of Ritalin. Although orally administered Ritalin is not strongly euphoriant, abusers have found other ways of administering the drug. The most common is to crush the Ritalin tablets and snort the powdered drug into the nose. The nasal cavity is richly endowed with blood vessels and, as with cocaine, the intranasal route provides a means of rapidly delivering drug to the blood-stream and brain. However, repeated use of this route leads to damage to the delicate intranasal membranes and inflammation as the tablet contains various other inert fillers that are not absorbed. This also makes intravenous injection hazardous, although some have used this route after dissolving the crushed tablets in water. There is little doubt that MP can be highly rewarding when administered by these routes—it is after all a member of the amphetamine family—and it is correctly classified as a Schedule II narcotic (Sannerud and Feussner 2000). In the USA, the DEA continues to issue warnings about the abuse potential of MP, but it is difficult to estimate how serious a problem this has become. More than 1000 emergency room visits for young people with MP intoxication are reported in the USA annually. One questionnaire among 6000 US high school students indicated that 13 per cent were taking illicit Ritalin, in many cases as a study aid. In normal people MP does have definite alerting and anti-fatigue effects. The children treated with psychostimulants may tend to want to continue using them when they become adolescents or college under-graduates and they no longer have a legitimate doctor's prescription. As one anonymous Harvard student put it:

> In all honesty, I haven't written a paper without Ritalin since my junior year in high school. I even wrote my Harvard essay on it. It keeps you up when you're tired, and makes you much more aware of what you're doing. Although there are certain risks involved, I think it's worth it.

Adderall is not immune from problems of abuse. According to a report from Texas, college students like Adderall because it allows them to stay awake all night for their studies:

> Adderall is going to react the same way with every person whether an individual needs it or not. It makes students stay awake and study because they take it at night—if you are prescribed Adderall, you are supposed to take it in the morn-ing—so ultimately Adderall is supposed to last a patient all day, but when stu-dents abuse it and take it at night, it makes them have the effects it would have had if they took it in the morning.

Judging by the number of US campus websites currently reporting Adderall abuse, this may be a growing trend among college students. They like Adderall because of its relatively long duration of action and the drug-induced heightening of concentration and alertness that it provides.

It is difficult to predict how this problem will grow. The situation in schools should become less acute with the increasing adoption of sustained-release formulations of Ritalin and Adderall. These allow once-daily dosing to be done at home, making it unnecessary for the school nurse to undertake the distribution of supplies of the drugs during the school day, and this should eventually make the school premises essentially drug free. The sustained-release preparations will also be impossible to abuse by snorting or injection as the active drug is trapped in an insoluble wax or resin matrix. However, currently the sustained-release drugs are very much more expensive and this may limit their adoption. The skin-patch formulation version of MP will make diversion to illicit use even more difficult or impossible. On the other hand, Ritalin and Adderall appear to be readily available 'with no hassle' from a variety of online pharmacies, making them easily obtainable. It is likely that among a generation of schoolchildren who have become accustomed to treatment with psychostimulants there will be many who will wish to continue such use into adolescence and adulthood. Others may find these drugs an easy way into the 'performance-enhancing' properties of the amphetamine class, and there will be yet others who abuse the drugs for their rewarding properties and become dependent upon them.

Society has learned to adjust to ADHD and the widespread use of psychostimulant drugs in many different ways. For example, it took some time and argument, but concessions were eventually won by advocates in the area of college athletics in the USA. The National College Athletic Association (NCAA) once prohibited Ritalin usage (as do the US and International Olympic Committees today) because of its 'possible acute performance-enhancing benefits'. In 1993, citing legal jeopardy as a reason for changing course, the NCAA capitulated. A letter from the team physician will suffice to allow an athlete to ingest Ritalin, even though that same athlete would be disqualified from participating in the Olympics if he were to test positive for stimulants.

In the field of higher education, where the first wave of Ritalin-taking children has now arrived, a diagnosis of ADHD can give entitlement to various types of special treatment. Students with ADHD can successfully demand extra time for various tests and examinations, or even for routine assignments. To refuse 'accommodation' is to risk a hornet's nest of liabilities, as a growing caseload shows. An article in *Forbes Magazine* in 1996 cited the example of Whittier Law School, which was sued by an ADHD-diagnosed student for giving only 20 extra minutes per hour-long examination instead of a full hour. The school, fearing an expensive legal battle, settled the suit.

A pharmacological advance has been the introduction of a new drug, atomoxetine (trade name Strattera), to treat the symptoms of ADHD. Atomoxetine does not belong to the amphetamine class and is not a scheduled narcotic. It acts as a selective inhibitor of the norepinephrine transporter in brain. It is too early to know whether atomoxetine will take over a large share of the ADHD market. It requires only once-daily dosing and it is not a stimulant drug; therefore it has little or no abuse potential. However, some clinical trials have suggested that although atomoxetine is efficacious in ADHD, it may be less effective than Adderall (Wigal *et al.* 2005).

The story of ADHD and its treatment with psychotropic drugs has been a remarkable one, awash with myths, critics, sceptics, pariahs, personal agendas, messiahs, enthusiasts, real science, and pseudoscience. I personally believe that Ritalin and Adderall have helped hundreds of thousands of children live more positive lives; it has saved them from educational under-achievement and lowered self-esteem and has relieved much family stress. To dismiss the potentially dramatic benefits of pharmacological treatment for ADHD risks withholding an effective treatment for a serious heritable behavioural disorder. In Europe, ADHD is still underdiagnosed and undertreated; we have much to learn from both the positive and the negative aspects of the Ritalin Age in the USA. On the other hand, the Ritalin Age has probably gone too far in the USA with overprescription of psychostimulants and some parents encouraging the use of such medicines for any badly behaved or academically underperforming child.

CHAPTER 4

Amphetamines as performance enhancers

'The idea of playing baseball without taking amphetamines or other stimulants is so absurd to some major leaguers that they have a catchphrase for it: 'playing naked'. There are of course varying degrees of nakedness; but the fact remains that popping pills—everything from caffeine tablets to Ritalin to the amphetamine capsules known as greenies or beans—is as standard to many ballplayers' pregame routine as stretching exercises and batting practice.'

(Verducci 2002)

4.1. Introduction

Almost as soon as Benzedrine became available in the USA, first as an inhaler in 1932 and then in pill form in 1936, people began to use it for non-medical reasons, simply to experience the euphoriant and stimulant effects. As described in more detail in Chapter 5, the casual misuse of orally administered amphetamines in the 1940s and 1950s evolved into the misuse of more dangerous forms of the drugs administered by injection, snorting, or smoking.

Amphetamines have long been used to enhance human performance. In this chapter we will review how they came to be used in the military and in sport, and still are widely used and abused.

4.2. Military uses

Ever since the 1930s, when they were first used in the Spanish Civil War, amphetamines have found an officially sanctioned use in the military to assist personnel in 'driving hard beyond the normal limits of human endurance'. The Second World War saw an enormous use of amphetamines by both sides in the conflict (Leake 1958; Grinspoon and Hedblom 1975).

In the 1930s, a private company in Berlin, named Temmler-Werke, which specialized in producing sedatives and neuroleptics, starting making methamphetamine which they called Pervitin. In 1938, Professor Ranke, who was head of the physiological institute of the newly founded Militärärztliche Akademie (Military Doctors' Academy) in Berlin, started testing Pervitin with the help of his students. During the war in Poland, a number of military doctors on duty there received large amounts of Pervitin to test under fighting conditions and to report on their experiences. They suggested that the pills should be given to pilots and drivers of trucks and tanks in particular. There followed widespread use of Pervitin by German troops to eliminate fatigue and increase physical endurance, and perhaps also to increase levels of aggression (Steinkamp 2003). It is possible that some of the excesses and atrocities committed by German soldiers were drug fuelled. However, it soon became clear that Pervitin could lead to heavy habitual use. Misuse was mainly a problem for military doctors, soldiers within the medical corps, and officers, especially those in staff positions. It was alleged that Adolf Hitler himself was a regular methamphetamine user throughout the Second World War (Heston and Heston 1979). In the early 1940s prescription of Pervitin was placed under the German opium laws, but it was still given to soldiers under medical control. There were severe punishments and even death sentences for crimes associated with Pervitin misuse. The most prominent misuser was the Luftwaffe General Ernst Udet (1896–1941) who later committed suicide (Keitel 1965).

In Japan, methamphetamine (known as Philopon, Wake-amine, or Hospitan) was used even more widely, almost compulsorily, among both military personnel and civilians working in the war effort. Statistics about the German and Japanese experience are hard to come by, but the British Armed Forces issued more than 70 million standard-dose D-amphetamine tablets, and American forces stationed in the UK during the 1940s had more than 100 million tablets available. After the war many soldiers returned home with an amphetamine habit—sanctioned by the military authorities! Monroe and Drell (1947) found that some 25 per cent of the prisoners in a US Army prison were abusers of Benzedrine inhalers, and most had probably been exposed to amphetamine through their previous army experience.

After the war the military use of amphetamine, far from declining, appeared to increase rapidly. During the Second World War amphetamines were used mainly by the Army for combat situations, by the Air Force for long flying missions, or by the Navy for sailors who needed to stay awake on watch at night, but by the time of the Korean War amphetamines had become general issue to US Army soldiers. A Congressional report (Select Committee on Crime 1971) noted that the US Navy had an active duty 'pill-per-person' annual requirement averaging 21 during the period 1966–1969; the Air Force requirement was 17.5 pills per person, and the Army requirement was 13.8. The total consumption of amphetamine by the US Armed Forces in this 4-year period, at 225 million tablets, exceeded the entire consumption by British and US forces during the Second World War! The use of amphetamines has since declined and they were temporarily banned by the US Air Force in 1992. However, they have recently been reintroduced during the Second Gulf War and its aftermath for both US and British Air Force combat missions. They are routinely used, for example, by US Air Force flight crews manning bomber flights from the USA to distant targets, where the duration of flights can be more than 24 hours. The US Air Force stresses that the use of amphetamine is voluntary, but there appears to be some element of coercion in the statement that pilots are required to sign:

> It has been explained to me and I understand that the US FDA had not approved the use of Dexedrine to manage fatigue . . . and I further understand that the decision to take the medication is mine alone.

But later on in the same consent form, pilots are informed that there are serious consequences to not taking the drug:

> Should I choose not to take it under circumstances where its use appears indicated . . . my commander, upon advice of the flight surgeon, may determine whether or not I should be considered unfit to fly a mission.

Nevertheless, not all pilots opt to take amphetamine. Kenagy *et al.* (2004) analysed the behaviour of 75 US Air Force B-2 bomber pilots flying a total of 94 combat missions from US bases to Iraq. The planes came from two alternative US bases, one involving a long (17 hours) and the other a very long (35 hours) mission. On the shorter mission 97 per cent of the pilots used D-amphetamine as opposed to taking short naps, but on the longer mission 94 per cent opted for naps and only 58 per cent took D-amphetamine.

The continuing use of D-amphetamine by the military remains controversial. Two US Air Force pilots were accused of involuntary manslaughter for an incident in which they dropped bombs on a Canadian unit engaged in a training mission in Afghanistan in 2002. Their defence attorney suggested that their judgement had been impaired as a result of amphetamine use on the mission (Bower 2003). However, the military use of amphetamines is likely to continue. With increasingly sophisticated night vision devices, for example, US forces will increasingly engage the enemy at night, when amphetamines may help to keep them awake and alert (Bower 2003).

4.3. Amphetamine abuse in sport

On a hot afternoon in 1967, an Englishman who had gone to France to make a living as a professional cyclist fell off his bicycle twice on Mont Ventoux in a strenuous part of the Tour de France and died in full view of the television cameras (Fig. 4.1). Tom Simpson, the greatest rider that the UK had ever produced, was 29. As Jacques Goddet, the Tour de France organizer, put it: 'It is not normal for an athlete of that age and in prime physical condition to die in such circumstances'. It was soon evident that amphetamine was a major factor in Tom

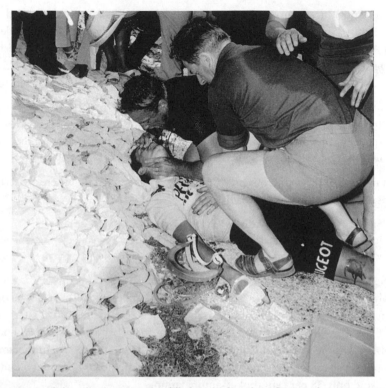

Figure 4.1 English cyclist Tom Simpson falls from his bicycle in the Tour de France 1967, and dies—with amphetamine as a factor.

Simpson's death. The drug was present in his blood and also in reserve supplies stashed in his pockets. He had drugged himself to climb the formidable mountain that rises above the plains of Provence. In the baking sun he had become overheated and dehydrated, and tumbled to his death (Fig. 4.1)

He was not the first cyclist to die from an amphetamine overdose. In the Olympic Games in Rome in 1960 the Danish cyclist Knut Jensen had fallen and died, and had also tested positive for amphetamine. The gruelling physical demands of long-distance cycling are very intense and dangerous. Competitors ride at speeds that no car driver would risk without a seatbelt and an airbag. Amphetamine, with its ability to help sustain long periods of mental/physical performance and attention, offers an obvious temptation. For many years amphetamines were widely used by competitors in the Tour de France and other long-distance cycle races. The Belgian cyclist Willy Voet described his first experience of taking amphetamine in the 1960s:

> Taking them was so simple. One pill half an hour before the start, the other halfway through the race. I went up to the registration table after I'd taken the

first pill. The hairs on my arms were standing up like porcupine quills and shivers were running up and down my body. The magic potion was working already. I was having to breathe deeply. The second the flag dropped I was off like a bullet from a gun. And I wasn't the only one. I was motoring—I was riding so fast that it scared me. I didn't feel hungry, but on the other hand I had a raging thirst throughout the whole race, which was a loop of about 120 kilometres. And I began to think I was a star! Fuelled by drugs I was able to keep up with guys who were physically stronger and better than me . . . All big names, and me the novice—I was the one telling them to get off their backsides and ride. As soon as they saw my face, they caught on. I must have had that look about me . . . The high lasted until about two laps from the finish. And then all of a sudden, it was if I had been knocked out. I hit the wall—I couldn't see or hear anything. If someone had walked into the road, I'd have ridden straight into them. I was left behind the lead group, but somehow managed to hold on to sixth place . . . . Of course this first try-out hadn't turned me into a winner, but I had felt as strong as an ox, and amphetamines keep calling you back for one more go. Curiosity was replaced by desire. (Voet 2002)

The introduction of compulsory drug testing in the 1980s helped to eradicate this dangerous practice, but the urge to use performance-enhancing drugs and to cheat the system was great. Voet became a *soigneur* to professional cycle teams, and in his book (Voet 2002) described the various tricks used to substitute a 'clean' urine sample for the real thing. Because of the tricks used to conceal 'clean' urine samples, cyclists eventually had to strip naked before producing a urine sample for test, but even then they found ingenious hiding places. Voet used one particularly effective technique.

> You have to get a rubber tube which is both flexible and rigid. At one end you fix a small cork, at the other a condom, running about a third of the way up the tube. Finally just as a precaution, you stick carpet pile, or any short hair, on the part of the tube which isn't in the condom.

> In the team car, when the rider comes to change before going to the drug control, you go on to stage two: you slip the part of the tube fitted with the condom up the backside, inject clean urine up the tube with a large syringe, cork it and stick it to the skin, following the line of the perineum, as far as the testicles. That's why the hairs are necessary, to hide the tube in case the doctor running the test decides to lean down. The condom full of urine is held in the anus, which has the advantage of keeping the urine at body temperature, so the doctor won't be suspicious, as he would be if presented with a flask of cold liquid. This system was never bettered— no doctor suspected a thing and I used it for three years without any worries. (Voet 2002)

Eventually, even this apparently foolproof system grew too well known and was abandoned. Nevertheless, the Tour de France continued to be plagued with drug scandals as cyclists found other performance-enhancing substances that were more difficult to detect.

Cycling was only one of many sports in which competitors sought to enhance their performance by taking amphetamines. Boxers and jockeys made use of the appetite-suppressant effects of amphetamines to keep their weight down, and some boxers used high doses to heighten their aggression and endurance. Some experiments were even made in dosing racehorses with amphetamine to improve their performance, although dosing the favourite horse with a barbiturate to slow it down proved more successful! The introduction of drug testing as a routine part of the Olympic competition is in large part due to the widespread use of amphetamines in many different sports arenas. But just how effective are amphetamines in enhancing performance? German laboratory experiments during the Second World War showed that injections of methamphetamine significantly increased the time that subjects could run on a treadmill before collapsing (Heyrodt and Weissenstein 1941). UK studies, more relevant to cyclists, showed that the performance of a normal subject on a cycle ergometer gradually diminished over a period of several hours, but amphetamine produced a marked rise in pedalling rate that could be maintained for some hours (Cuthbertson and Knox 1947). Other studies showed that soldiers given amphetamine were able to march long distances, and were willing to continue marching even with severe foot blisters (Tyler 1947; reviewed by Laties and Weiss 1981).

Amphetamine-induced increases in endurance can also be seen in laboratory animals: D-amphetamine increased the length of time that rats ran in a treadmill before failing to keep up with its rate (Gerald 1978), and the swimming performance of rats could also be prolonged by amphetamine (Bhagat and Wheeler 1973).

The most systematic study of the effects of amphetamine on athletic performance was undertaken at the request of the American Medical Association's Committee on Amphetamine Drugs and Athletes by Gene Smith and Henry Beecher at Harvard in the 1950s (Smith and Beecher 1959). At their annual convention in 1957 the American Medical Association denounced the increasing prevalence of amphetamine abuse by athletes and some coaches and established this committee to investigate. Smith and Beecher performed six different experiments involving college athletes (swimmers, runners, shot putters, and weight lifters). The trials were double-blinded and placebo-controlled, with the same subjects studied on four 'amphetamine days' and four 'placebo days' for comparison. Neither subjects nor investigators knew whether drug or placebo was given on any particular day. The results were not dramatic but they were very clear cut. All classes of athletes performed better under the influence of amphetamine (14 mg per 70 kg body weight). Eighty-five per cent of the weight throwers, 63–97 per cent of swimmers, and 73 per cent of the runners performed better under the influence of amphetamine than with placebo. The effects were small but statistically significant. The weight throwers gained the maximum benefit from amphetamine (3–4 per cent); runners obtained an improvement of approximately 1.5 per cent and swimmers an improvement of around 1 per cent. These are small effects, but in the highly competitive world of athletics can make the difference between winning and losing. The studies showed unequivocally that the performance of highly trained fit athletes can be improved significantly by amphetamine.

Amphetamine use became embedded in many different sports. It entered professional football in the USA after the Second World War and remained for decades thereafter. A fascinating study of how footballers used amphetamine was provided by Arnold Mandell, a Professor of Psychiatry at the University of California in San Diego (Mandell 1976; Mandell et al. 1981). He acted as the 'psychological coach' to the San Diego Chargers, a national league professional football team, for some years and was able to observe at first hand the behaviour of the players and also to observe other professional football teams. During the period 1968–1969 bulk drug purchase records for the San Diego team showed that an average of 60–70 mg of amphetamine was used per man for each game. During the 1973 season Mandell was able to work with the team directly. Before games he often observed the sudden emergence in some players of uncharacteristic obscenities, violent diarrhoea and vomiting, white lips, temper tantrums, and repetitive pacing with stereotyped gestures. Players used the drug to counteract pain, 'to get calmed down', and 'to get psyched up'. An interesting pattern of task-related dose selection was observed according to the different positions that players occupied in the field. Those in skilled positions (quarterbacks, wide receivers, running backs) took small doses of amphetamine (5–10 mg) in the belief that it would improve their energy and creative performance. Players in defensive positions (linebackers and offensive linesmen) took somewhat higher doses (15–45 mg) in the belief that they would become fearless and stable in defence, and the heavy end of the team (defensive end, defensive tackle) took high doses (50–200 mg) to induce a manic high, sometimes accompanied by paranoiac rage. The latter doses are comparable to those used by 'speed freaks' and it is highly questionable that they could have improved the footballers' performance. Behaviour after such large doses of amphetamine tends to become stereotyped, and players often had difficulty in adjusting their play, disregarding signals from other team members. However, according to Mandell, the footballers' use of amphetamine was usually a once-weekly exposure, and was not associated with dependence and addiction. Although amphetamine use in professional football has shifted from open jars of pills available to all before the game to physicians willing to prescribe discretely, the behaviour is firmly engrained. Mandell wrote a book about his experiences, *The Nightmare Season* (Mandell 1976). However, after a State of California Medical Board review in

1977 he was found guilty of improperly prescribing amphetamines and placed on probation for 5 years, with his right to prescribe stimulants suspended; however, he retained his medical license.

Few sports have been immune from amphetamine misuse. Amphetamines are said to have a long tradition in US professional baseball (Verducci 2002). Some say that amphetamine use is more widespread than steroid use in a sport where players are ground down by playing 162 games over 183 days during the regular season, with constant travel and all-night flights leaving many weary. Despite these allegations, amphetamines were left untouched by baseball's 2004 drug-testing agreement, with the issue left for the sport's medical advisers to study. As one journalist put it:

> Major-league players are applauding baseball's new steroid policy, some of them with great sincerity. Behind the scenes, however, there is a great sense of relief. Amphetamines remain fair game . . . For all of the benefits gained by steroids, from strength to bat speed to increased aggressiveness, the flip side can bring deteriorating health and counterproductive mood swings. Many have tried steroids, only to be run out of sports by the side effects. Amphetamines are no bargain, health-wise, but the formula is much simpler: Stay alert, perform better. Say it's around midnight near the end of an exhausting road trip. If you're looking for a key hit against someone throwing 100 mph gas, there's no comparison between a tired, drowsy ballplayer and a guy so jacked-up, mentally, he steps to the plate with a wide-eyed vengeance. (Bruce Jenkins, *San Francisco Chronicle*, 15 January 2005)

....

CHAPTER 5

Illicit amphetamine use around the world

Benzedrine sulphate thus becomes one more example of a drug which is useful in a limited field of therapeutics but which has been diverted to uncontrolled use by the public for related but not similar purposes.

(JAMA 1937)

5.1. Introduction

A United Nations report (United Nations 2003) estimated a worldwide total of 34 million people who regularly abuse amphetamine-like stimulants and 8 million who use ecstasy. This exceeds the number of heroin and cocaine abusers combined. D-Amphetamine and D-methamphetamine are among the most widely used of all illicit drugs, ranking second in popularity only to cannabis in many countries. It is now generally recognized that the amphetamines are drugs of addiction, and in this chapter we will review the evidence for this and explore the underlying brain mechanisms. The social history of amphetamine abuse in various parts of the world is also reviewed.

5.2. Are amphetamines addictive? Human experience

For several decades after the introduction of amphetamines as medicines it was widely believed that they were not addictive. Since it is now clear that this was wrong, how did this happen? The answer seems to be that physicians and psychiatrists thought of 'addiction' in terms of what they knew about heroin and other opiates. In these cases addiction was clearly defined by the very obvious physical withdrawal syndrome that users experienced when drug use was stopped. These included severe gastrointestinal upsets, vomiting, pain, and diarrhoea, with sweating and sometimes physical convulsions. Heroin withdrawal is painful and can be life-threatening. Since no such obvious physical withdrawal was seen when regular users of amphetamine stopped taking the drug, it was wrongly concluded that there was no addiction.

In a report produced in 1957 the WHO Expert Committee on Addiction-Producing Drugs attempted to distinguish between 'drug addiction' and 'drug habituation, (habit)' as representing different grades of a scale, but 'drug addiction' still required some degree of physical dependence (Grinspoon and Hedblom 1975). The WHO Expert Committee later suggested a new term, 'drug dependence', to cover all forms of compulsive drug-taking, and they defined 'drug dependence of amphetamine type' (WHO 1964). The characteristics included the following.

1. A desire or need to continue taking the drug.

2. Consumption of increasing amounts to obtain greater excitatory and euphoric effects or to combat fatigue, accompanied in some measure by the development of tolerance.

3. A psychic dependence on the effects of the drug related to a subjective and individual appreciation of the drug's effects.

4. General absence of physical dependence so that there is no characteristic abstinence syndrome when the drug is discontinued.

This was an important step forward in defining what was beginning to be recognized as a serious problem in the use of amphetamines. It satisfied to some extent the wishes of the American Medical Association (and presumably the manufacturers of amphetamines) to avoid using the word 'addiction' in the context of amphetamines (American Medical Association 1963).

On the ground the problem was becoming clearer. In the UK the authors of a study of amphetamine abuse in Newcastle upon Tyne stated that, in their view, a considerable abuse of amphetamines existed, and that habituation and addiction occurred frequently. They commented in respect to the WHO 1957 definition of addiction that:

> It must be conceded that a number of patients taking excessive quantities of
> amphetamine fulfil this definition. They certainly suffer an overpowering desire
> to continue taking the drug, they take it in amounts far exceeding the usual
> therapeutic dose, they may be prepared to break the law to obtain supplies, they
> are dependent upon it, and they sometimes become psychotic. Furthermore,
> withdrawal symptoms may occur, notably states of depression in which suicide
> may occur. (Kiloh and Brandon 1962)

Of course, not all regular users of amphetamines become dependent on the drug. Millions of adults and children have used the drugs medically without this happening, and large numbers of people have taken amphetamines to enhance performance—in the military, in sports, and in the many other ways in which these drugs have been casually employed—in most cases without suffering adverse effects or dependence. Angrist and Sudilvosky (1978) suggested a distinction between 'low-dose non-medical stimulant use' and 'high-dose non-medical stimulant use', and argued that it is the use of high doses of amphetamines that distinguishes drug abuse and dependence. Although it is hard to draw such a distinct line between categories of amphetamine users, the authors argued that high-dose use differed from low-dose use in that dependence was more severe and in that the dose was escalated. The resulting high doses were incompatible with normal functioning, and carried with them liabilities of toxicity, severely disturbed behaviour, dysphoria, and psychosis.

Although high doses of orally administered amphetamine can lead to dependence, there is little doubt that the route of administration is also very important. The rapidity and intensity of onset of the drug effect after intravenous injection or smoking increase the rate and strength of development of psychological dependence. The 'rush' or 'flash' following such rapid routes of administration has often been described as a 'whole body orgasm' and is highly prized (Smith and Fischer 1970) (see Chapter 3). However, as the 'rush' declines, restlessness, nervousness, and agitation replace nirvana. Irritability progresses to paranoia, fatigue, and depression as the ride comes to an end. The urge to repeat the drug experience is often irresistible. The intensity of the rush is dose related (Jönsson et al. 1969) and so users tend to administer ever higher doses. Moreover, the desire to re-experience the rush may lead to a cycle of additional doses and increasing overall cumulative dose. This type of stimulant use is known as 'speeding' and is particularly common in methamphetamine abusers ('speed freaks'). A 'run' can last for several days at a time, during which the user is unable to eat or sleep until he 'crashes' into a deep sleep that can last for 18 h. Repeated speeding can lead to cycles of unproductive frenzied activity, stereotyped behaviour known as punding (see Chapter 2), or psychosis (see Chapter 6), alternating with exhaustion, extended sleep, and subsequent dysphoric lethargy. Loss of appetite may become anorexia, a state in which the user finds it difficult to eat at all, resulting in extreme and debilitating weight loss. Repeated cycles of speeding can lead to a severe form of dependence and a complete preoccupation with the drug and its effects. The distressing features of the crash after an amphetamine binge were described by Grinspoon and Hedblom (1975):

> The 'crashing' amphetamine abuser lacks the energy to complain and may seem to be merely exhausted and in need of sleep. Recently investigators have looked more closely, and the emerging picture is unpleasant and painful. Extreme lethargy and fatigue are almost invariably reported. Although the 'crasher' may sleep for several days, he never sleeps well, and often wakes screaming from nightmares. On awakening, he may experience anxiety attacks and suicidally severe depression. His psychic disruption and loss of self control may lead to violent acting out of sexual conflicts and aggressive impulses. He often experiences acute fear and terror and is as likely to turn homicidal as suicidal. He is apt to be extremely irritable and demanding, driving people away just when he most needs their help. His head aches; he may have trouble breathing; he sweats profusely; his body is racked by alternating sensations of extreme heat and cold

and distressing muscle cramps. He may feel so exhausted that he is unable even to stand. He is characteristically constipated, and suffers painful gastrointestinal cramps.

One methamphetamine user in California offered this very articulate description:

> There's a certain pattern . . . Your first day off you're okay because the stuff is still kicking in your system so you don't feel the high that you did but you don't feel the down that your going to. On the second day, you become a zombie, some Haitian voodoo doctor's idea of a good human being! . . . You're an eating and sleeping machine! You get what we call the 'waking nods'! Third day is even worse, it's the absolute coma. The only time that you wake up are the times you want to eat! Fourth day, same thing! It's kind of a mimic of the second day, you're a zombie . . . You have no motivation; you don't have a terrible desire to do the drug because you know it won't work on you! Fifth day, you start to wake up . . . You get a glimmer of your real self back and that's the time you start again! Go back out and find some and you do it and boom, you're right back up to where you were. (Morgan and Beck 1997)

How did we ever believe that amphetamine abuse was not associated with physical dependence and withdrawal?

Scientific evidence for a withdrawal effect on sleep patterns was provided by Oswald and Thacore (1963) who studied regular amphetamine users in a sleep laboratory, making electrical recordings from their scalp of their sleep patterns. They found that during amphetamine use the subjects slept for normal periods of time but the period spent in the dreaming state (rapid eye movement (REM) sleep) was reduced. Conversely, on withdrawal of the drug there was a significant rebound, with abnormally long periods spent in REM sleep. The findings were one of the first to describe evidence of physical withdrawal.

As with the rebound seen in REM sleep, amphetamine abusers often experience an increase in appetite during withdrawal, awakening voraciously hungry after a binge (Kramer 1969).

International agreement on definitions was reached with the advent of DSM-IV-TR (American Psychiatric Association 2000) which now uses the term 'substance dependence'. The criteria for substance dependence are defined as follows (American Psychiatric Association 2000).

> A maladaptive pattern of substance abuse, leading to clinically significant impairment or distress, as manifested by three (or more) of the following, occurring at any time in the same 12-month period:
> 1. Tolerance, as defined by either of the following:
>   a) A need for markedly increased amount of the substance to achieve intoxication or desired effect.
>   b) Markedly diminished effect with continued use of the same amount of the substance.

2. Withdrawal, as defined by either of the following:
   a) the characteristic withdrawal syndrome for the substance
   b) the same (or a closely related) substance is taken to relieve or avoid with-
      drawal symptoms.
3. The substance is often taken in larger amounts or over a longer period than
   was intended.
4. There is a persistent desire or unsuccessful efforts to cut down or control
   substance use.
5. A great deal of time is spent in activities necessary to obtain the substance
   (e.g. visiting multiple doctors or driving long distances), use the substance
   (e.g. chain-smoking), or recover from its effects.
6. Important social, occupational, or recreational activities are given up or
   reduced because of substance use.
7. The substance use is continued despite knowledge of having a persistent or
   recurrent physical or psychological problem that is likely to have been caused or
   exacerbated by the substance (e.g. current cocaine use despite recognition of
   cocaine-induced depression or continued drinking despite recognition that an
   ulcer was made worse by alcohol consumption).

Substance dependence with physiological dependence is diagnosed if there is evidence of tolerance or withdrawal.

Substance dependence without physiological dependence is diagnosed if there is
no evidence of tolerance or withdrawal.

The DSM-IV classification also recognizes a lesser form of maladaptive
pattern of drug use termed 'substance abuse'. This describes drug use that has
recurrent and significant adverse consequences, but does not include tolerance,
withdrawal or a pattern of compulsive use. The DSM-IV criteria for substance
abuse are as follows.

A. A maladaptive pattern of substance use leading to clinically significant
   impairment of distress, as manifested by one (or more) of the following,
   occurring within a 12-month period:
   Recurrent substance use resulting in a failure to fulfil major role obligations at
   work, school, or home (e.g. repeated absences or poor work performance
   related to substance use; substance-related absences, suspensions, or expulsions
   from school; neglect of children or household).
   Recurrent substance use in situations in which it is physically hazardous (e.g.
   driving an automobile or operating a machine when impaired by substance use).
   Recurrent substance-related legal problems (e.g. arrests for substance-related
   conduct).
   Continued substance use despite having persistent or recurrent social or interpersonal problems caused or exacerbated by the effects of the substance (e.g.
   arguments with spouse about consequences of intoxication, physical fights).

B. The symptoms have never met the criteria for substance-dependence for this
   class of substance.

Amphetamine abuse can lead to both substance dependence and the less severe, but still seriously damaging, substance abuse.

5.3. What are the brain mechanisms that underlie amphetamine dependence/addiction?

It is clear that some amphetamine users do become dependent on the drug, but what are the brain mechanisms that underlie this phenomenon? In order to answer that question we need to consider more generally the advances in scientific understanding of the neurobiology of drug dependence.

All drugs capable of causing dependence share certain common features. They are readily self-administered by experimental animals. This in turn must mean that the drug acts as a 'positive reinforcer', i.e. it has some rewarding or pleasurable property. Amphetamines are no exception; both monkeys and rats can be trained to self-administer these drugs. Usually this involves training the animals to press a lever to self-inject a small dose intravenously. For example, Sannerud et al. (1989) trained baboons to self-inject a variety of amphetamines, having first accustomed the animals to the procedure by allowing them to self-administer cocaine. The animals were allowed access to the drugs every 3 h, signalled by a light. They had to press a lever more than 100 times in order to obtain a drug injection. The animals showed a dose-dependent increase in lever pressing to obtain drug injections when offered a variety of amphetamines. D-Amphetamine itself gave the most robust effects, but the animals also self-administered a variety of amphetamine analogues used as appetite suppressants, including phentermine, diethylpropion, phenmetrazine, benzphetamine, and chlorphentermine. Amphetamines are very powerful reinforcers in animals trained to self-administer them. If monkeys are given unrestricted access, they will overdose on amphetamine or methamphetamine to the exclusion of all other behaviour. In one study all the monkeys given free access to D-amphetamine or methamphetamine died within a week (Johanson et al. 1976).

Addiction can be viewed as an aberrant form of reinforcement learning (Volkow and Li 2004). At its most basic level, reinforcement learning is the ability to lean to act on the basis of important outcomes such as reward or punishment. The idea of 'motivational state' is important in considering reinforcement learning. Natural motivations such as hunger or thirst are important determinants of behaviour. For example, a hungry animal will seek food, but a sated animal will not. In the case of drug addiction, drug craving represents an unnatural motivational state. Drug addiction manifests as a compulsive drive to take a drug despite serious adverse consequences. This aberrant behaviour has traditionally been viewed as a bad 'choice' that is made voluntarily by the addict. However, recent studies have shown that repeated drug use leads to long-lasting changes in the brain that undermine voluntary control.

An important discovery made in the 1950s was that if minute electrodes are implanted in certain regions in the brain, animals can be taught to self-stimulate to receive small pulses of electrical stimulation (Olds and Milner 1954). Such intracranial self-stimulation (ICSS) behaviour appears to plug directly into the brain circuits of reward and pleasure normally activated during reinforcement learning. Later, it became apparent that the regions of the brain which sustain ICSS correspond to those containing ascending neural tracts which originate in the brainstem and whose fibres innervate many structures in the forebrain limbic system which is known to be associated with emotional behaviour and with reward and pleasure. The neurotransmitter dopamine is particularly well represented in the ICSS tracts.

A major advance in understanding was the realization that the dopamine system in the brain plays an important role in the rewarding properties of all drugs of abuse, not just those such as the amphetamines and cocaine which act directly to promote dopamine release, but others, such as nicotine, heroin, cannabis, and alcohol, which do not activate dopamine mechanisms directly but which are able indirectly to stimulate dopamine release in the brain (Koob et al. 1998; Di Chiara et al. 2004; Volkow and Li 2004).

Furthermore, these drugs share an ability to stimulate dopamine release in specific brain regions. The neuronal systems that utilize dopamine as their neurotransmitter are organized in two main pathways in the brain: a dorsally located pathway from the brainstem to the basal ganglia, in which dopamine plays an important role in coordinating voluntary movements, and a ventral pathway arising from the brainstem and projecting forwards to various regions of the limbic system. The ability of drugs of abuse to trigger dopamine release in one small ventrally placed dopamine-rich region of the limbic system, the shell region of the nucleus accumbens, appears to be critical in determining the addictive potential of these drugs. The precise function of dopamine release in this and other regions of the brain remains unclear, but one hypothesis is that dopamine release in the nucleus accumbens represents a natural mechanism normally triggered by pleasurable stimuli in the environment, such as palatable food, sex, water, etc (Ungless 2004). The release of dopamine by such stimuli may act as a 'teaching signal' in a mechanism whereby the animal learns to seek rewarding environmental events again in the future. The ability of psychoactive drugs to trigger this natural mechanism, and to cause the animal or human to seek further doses of the drug, could be viewed as an aberrant form of learning, where the drug 'hijacks' a natural mechanism in the brain, leading eventually to drug dependence (Everitt et al. 2001; Di Chiara et al. 2004; Volkow and Li 2004).

Brain imaging allows us to study which brain regions are selectively activated by amphetamines. Völlm et al. (2004) used MRI to study the effects of a low dose of intravenous methamphetamine (0.15 mg/kg) versus placebo in drug-naive volunteers. They found highly selective and localized activations of brain activity in the medial orbitofrontal cortex, the anterior cingulate cortex, and the ventral striatum, all regions believed to represent key parts of 'reward circuitry'.

The conclusion that drug-induced dopamine release in the nucleus accumbens shell region is critical in determining drug dependence emerged from many different types of experimental evidence. Placing minute cannulae into the brain of an experimental animal makes it possible to collect and measure released chemicals. In this way it was possible to measure directly amphetamine-induced dopamine release in the nucleus accumbens shell region, and to show that this occurred selectively in that brain region in response to various drugs of abuse (Di Chiara *et al.* 2004). Conversely, selective lesions of the dopamine system in the nucleus accumbens caused by local microinjections of the dopamine neurotoxin 6-hydroxydopamine (see Chapter 2) eliminated the propensity of animals to self-administer these drugs. Similar effects were seen after the local administration of dopamine antagonist drugs into the nucleus accumbens (Koob *et al.* 1998).

Although dopamine release plays a key role in determining drug-seeking behaviour, it is not thought to represent the 'pleasure' signal *per se* although its release may correlate with activity in other systems that do (Berridge and Robinson 1998). One hypothesis is that the pleasurable aspects of reward are mediated not by dopamine but via activation of the naturally occurring opiate (morphine-like) system in the brain (Everitt *et al.* 2001).

A further complication in understanding the role of dopamine in drug dependence is that dopamine neurons appear to fire in two different modes, known as 'tonic' and 'phasic' (Grace 2000). In the tonic mode neurons fire slowly, giving rise to low levels of dopamine both in the regions associated with synaptic contacts with other cells and in non-synaptic regions. This contrasts with phasic firing, which occurs in bursts of impulses and gives rise to a 'spike' in dopamine release, particularly important in activating post-synaptic neurons. The ability of intravenously administered or smoked drugs to mimic this phasic release of dopamine may help to explain why such routes of drug administration are more likely to lead to drug dependence. The slow absorption of orally administered drugs cannot mimic phasic dopamine release, but may only be capable of simulating the tonic mode of dopamine release, which is not in itself adequate to lead to subsequent dependence. This may explain, for example, why smoked methamphetamine is highly addictive, whereas orally administered Ritalin (methylphenidate) is not (see Chapter 3). Samaha and Robinson (2005) argued that rapidly administered drugs are addictive because they are able to engage limbic system circuits involved in neurobehavioural plasticity.

But how does the repeated drug-induced release of dopamine in the brain lead to a chronic condition of drug dependence? How is the dopamine 'teaching signal' interpreted? Clearly, what is going on represents a series of lasting changes in brain function. The exact molecular mechanisms underlying these changes are still poorly understood, but the development of dependence is believed to be due to drug-induced changes in gene expression in the brain. Nestler (2004) has focused on two genes in particular whose expression is altered in the nucleus accumbens in response to the repeated administration of various drugs of abuse. Both genes encode for proteins known as 'transcription factors' which, in turn, are involved in regulating the expression of other genes. One gene, known as *CREB*, appears to be intimately involved in those aspects of dependence underlying the withdrawal syndrome—the emergence of a negative emotional state (unhappiness, anxiety, irritability) when access to the drug is denied which is a key feature of dependence and which reinforces continuing drug-taking behaviour. A second transcription factor gene, known as *ΔFosB*, appears to be associated with sensitization to drug exposure and may be associated with increased drive and motivation or craving for the drug, which is also a key element of dependence.

5.4. Are there pharmacological differences between amphetamine and methamphetamine?

An intriguing question is whether there are differences between the mode of action of amphetamine and methamphetamine which might explain the generally accepted view that methamphetamine is more potent and more addictive than amphetamine. The 'epidemics' of amphetamine abuse witnessed in the post-war period in Japan and the USA, and now in South East Asia, have all involved methamphetamine rather than D-amphetamine. The US National Institute of Drug Abuse describes methamphetamine as a 'potent and highly addictive form of amphetamine'—but is there any evidence to substantiate this?

One hypothesis is that methamphetamine is a somewhat more potent psychostimulant than amphetamine but at the same time its peripheral sympathomimetic effects (e.g. heart rate, blood pressure) are less prominent because it is less potent than amphetamine in inhibiting the norepinephrine transporter in sympathetic nerves. This means that methamphetamine users can safely take higher doses of methamphetamine than would be tolerated for amphetamine, leading to a higher propensity for abuse. However, there is little evidence that methamphetamine is significantly more potent as a psychostimulant. Animals self-administer both drugs at comparable doses and rates (Balster and Schuster 1973) and humans prefer similar doses (Martin *et al.* 1971). Indeed, human users cannot distinguish one drug from the other when they are given acutely (Lamb and Henningfield 1994). Furthermore, a direct comparison of the ability of the two drugs to stimulate locomotor activity in rats failed to show any

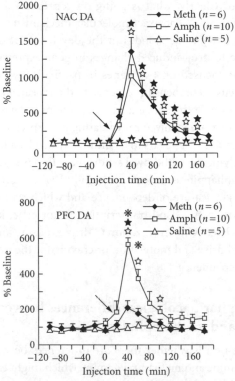

Figure 5.1 Effect of an injection of 2 mg/kg of amphetamine (Amph) or methamphetamine (Meth) on dopamine (DA) release in two regions of rat brain: the nucleus accumbens (NAC) and the prefrontal cortex (PFC). Results are mean values from 6–10 experiments. The time of injection is indicated by time zero. Filled star, methamphetamine data point statistically significant ($P < 0.05$) from baseline; open star, amphetamine data point statistically significant ($P < 0.05$) from baseline. *Statistically significant difference between methamphetamine and amphetamine data points. (Reproduced from J.R. Shoblock *et al.*, *Psychopharmacology*, **165**, 359–369, 2003.)

significant differences in potency (Shoblock *et al.* 2003). However, these authors did find some potentially important differences in the ability of the two drugs to promote dopamine release in different regions of the rat brain. Using implanted cannulas, they were able to show that both amphetamine and methamphetamine caused very significant increases in dopamine release in the nucleus accumbens (about 10-fold over baseline), as expected. However, in another region of brain, the prefrontal cortex, amphetamine was much more effective than methamphetamine in stimulating dopamine release (Fig. 5.1). This difference could be very significant in behavioural terms. Whereas dopamine release in the nucleus accumbens is acknowledged as a major mediator of drug reinforcement, in the prefrontal cortex it may, in contrast, be related to inhibition of reward

(Tzschentke and Schmidt 2000). Thus, while dopamine antagonist drugs administered into the nucleus accumbens reduce reward, the same drugs injected into the prefrontal cortex enhance reward (Duvauchelle *et al.* 1992). Similarly, dopamine-mimetic drugs have opposite effects on reward when injected into the nucleus accumbens or the prefrontal cortex (Olds 1990). Thus, by activating dopamine release in both the nucleus accumbens and in the prefrontal cortex, amphetamine may activate pathways that tend to counteract the rewarding effects of the drug, making it less likely to lead to dependence (Shoblock *et al.* 2003).

But why does amphetamine differ from methamphetamine in its ability to promote dopamine release in the prefrontal cortex, as both drugs potently interact with the dopamine transporter and dopamine storage mechanisms? The answer may lie in the unexpected finding that the dopamine transporter is relatively sparsely present in the dopamine nerves in the prefrontal cortex (Sesack *et al.* 1998). Dopamine appears to be inactivated in this brain region not by uptake into dopamine nerves via the dopamine transporter, but by uptake into adjacent norepinephrine-containing nerves via the norepinephrine transporter, for which dopamine is a good substrate (see Table 3.1) (Morón *et al.* 2002). Because amphetamine is a more potent inhibitor of the norepinephrine transporter than methamphetamine, it is more effective than methamphetamine in promoting increases in dopamine in the prefrontal cortex. Whether this is the correct pharmacological explanation remains to be confirmed, but clearly there are some subtle differences in the actions of the two drugs in the brain.

Another difference observed by Shoblock *et al.* (2003) was that, whereas amphetamine provoked an increase in glutamate release in the nucleus accumbens, methamphetamine did not. It has been suggested that increased glutamate levels in the nucleus accumbens have an inhibiting effect on reward mechanisms.

A physicochemical feature that may help to explain the current vogue for smoked methamphetamine ('ice') is that methamphetamine hydrochloride can be volatilized at temperatures that do not cause chemical degradation, whereas the common form of amphetamine (D-amphetamine sulphate) cannot; it needs to be heated to more than 300 °C to volatilize and at that temperature it is degraded. However, this alone cannot explain the current popularity of methamphetamine. Smoking appears to have become a favoured route for administering the drug, but only about 50 per cent of methamphetamine users employ this route and there are large geographical differences in the methods used. In 2000–2001 smoking accounted for more than 50 per cent of all use in San Diego, California, but in Texas more than 50 per cent of methamphetamine users injected the drug, and in Minneapolis–St Paul sniffing was the preferred route (http://www.drug-rehabs.com/methamphetamines-rehab.htm).

5.5. A social history of amphetamine abuse

5.5.1. Amphetamines in the USA

Early history

Almost as soon as Benzedrine became available in tablet form it began to be used for non-medical purposes. One of the first reported examples of Benzedrine misuse occurred among students at the University of Minnesota and was described in an Editorial in the *Journal of the American Medical Association* in 1937:

> Tablets of benzedrine sulfate were used in the department of psychology at the University of Minnesota for the purpose of determining its effects in mental efficiency tests. It was noted that the drug prevented sleepiness and 'pepped up' the person who was fatigued. Apparently this information was disseminated to the student body by word of mouth and the drug has been and still is being obtained by the students from drug stores for purpose of avoiding sleep and fatigue when preparing for examinations. (JAMA 1937)

It was unfortunate that the authors of this editorial incautiously used the term 'pep pills' to describe Benzedrine, no doubt making it even more attractive to students and other potential users. A report from the Maudsley Hospital, London, that Benzedrine caused quite marked increases in scores on intelligence tests (Sargent and Blackburn 1936) may have further enhanced the attractiveness of the drug to students. However, the British study was conducted in populations of hospitalized psychiatric patients, and such effects on IQ were not seen subsequently in normal subjects (see Chapter 2). Smith Kline and French, the manufacturers of Benzedrine, must have had some misgivings about the sudden popularity of their drug, as they sent a letter to US physicians suggesting some caution in its use (American Medical Association 1937). At that time Benzedrine was freely available over the counter in the USA; it did not become a prescription drug until 1939. However, even after that there were many approved medical uses and it remained easy to obtain (Chapter 3). Ever since 1937 students around the world have used amphetamine as a late-night 'pick-me-up' to keep studying for their examinations. The modern-day versions currently in vogue on US campuses for this use are Adderall and Ritalin, intended for the treatment of ADHD (Chapter 3).

After the introduction of the Benzedrine inhaler people soon discovered that the rather large amount of DL-amphetamine that these contained (250 mg, equivalent to 50 doses of a 5-mg pill) could fairly easily be extracted after breaking the inhaler open. The cotton strips impregnated with amphetamine in free-base oil form were folded into eight pieces, each of which when torn off conveniently represented a substantial dose of around 30 mg Benzedrine. The drug could be dissolved in coffee or alcohol, or the cotton strips inside could be chewed or simply swallowed whole. A classic study of the inmates of the US Military Prison at Fort Harrison, Indiana, shortly after the Second World War revealed that about a quarter of them confessed to this form of amphetamine abuse (Monroe and Drell 1947). Inhaler abuse became quite widespread in the USA, although Benzedrine was also easily available to the general public in pill form. The caution printed on the Benzedrine inhaler, 'Warning! For inhalation only! Unfit for internal use! Dangerous if swallowed!', was about as much use as the similar injunction plastered on bottles of surgical spirit during the prohibition era or the warnings printed on cigarette packets! Long after the Benzedrine inhaler was withdrawn from sale, inhaler misuse continued in other ways. Greenberg and Lustig (1966) described the misuse of the Dristan inhaler (which contained 250 mg of the amphetamine analogue mephentermine) in another US military prison. One of the inmates described the habit as follows:

> Some like it 'cause it's a cheap kick when they can't get nothing else, and some just like it. It's an easy thing; you can get it anywhere, in your friendly neighbourhood drugstore, man . . . And if you get picked up, so there's an inhaler in your pocket and you got a bad cold, they can't do anything to you for that, can they?

The post-war era of tolerance

The non-medical use of amphetamines spread rapidly in the 20 years after the Second World War. This was partly due to the attitude of the medical community to these drugs, which continued to view them as safe and effective medicines, and partly due to the widespread exposure of US military personnel to D-amphetamine during the war.

Most people viewed Benzedrine as a harmless stimulant. Harry 'The Hipster' Gibson, a pianist and singer who went in for swinging jazz with surreal lyrics, had a hit with his 1940s song *Who Put the Benzedrine in Mrs Murphy's Ovaltine*:

> 'Mrs Murphy couldn't sleep, her legs were slightly off the beat
> Until she solved her problems with a can of Ovaltine
> She drank a couple every night
> Ooh-Aah! How she did dream!
> But something rough got into that stuff, and made her neighbours scream
> 'Who put the Benzedrine in Mrs Murphy's Ovaltine?'
> Where did she get that stuff, now she can't get enough?'

Nevertheless, the dangers of abuse and addiction had been warned of early on. Reifenstein and Davidoff (1939), in their otherwise enthusiastic review of the medical uses of Benzedrine, noted:

> We are convinced that in certain persons at least, benzedrine sulphate is habit-forming. We have noticed this tendency in individuals addicted to alcohol, morphine and other drugs, in neurotic persons who crave medication, and in people who work under excessive strain such as actors, students, nurses and physicians.

Waud (1938) first reported the cardiovascular toxicity of high doses of Benzedrine, and also warned:

> The question of addiction to Benzedrine is not settled but I believe the possibility is not to be treated lightly, for most drugs that produce a pleasant effect on the brain (either stimulating or quieting in nature) have their addicts.

But on the whole these warning were ignored. Most physicians shared the view expressed in an Editorial on Benzedrine published in the *British Medical Journal* in 1939:

> The much-discussed question of habit formation has not yet been settled, but the danger does not appear to be serious. (BMJ 1939)

Perhaps the reason why most physicians did not view amphetamines as likely to cause addiction was because they had a limited view of addiction, referring to morphine/heroin, with the associated violent physical withdrawal syndrome. No such withdrawal was seen when amphetamine use stopped, and the importance of 'craving' in the description of drug dependence was not clearly recognized at that time (Angrist and Sudilovsky 1978).

The experience of an epidemic of methamphetamine abuse in Japan following the Second World War (see below), with clear evidence of addiction and tolerance in many users, should have served as a warning, but it was largely unknown to physicians in the West. In the period 1945–1958 only a handful of cases of amphetamine dependence were reported in the Western medical literature (Angrist and Sudilovsky 1978).

During the 1950s and 1960s the medical use of amphetamines grew rapidly, mainly as appetite suppressants. However, non-medical uses also expanded enormously. Amphetamine was widely used by people of all classes as a universal 'pick-me-up'. In a book published in 1958, an eminent Professor of Pharmacology at Ohio State University extolled the medical virtues of amphetamine for a variety of illnesses. He testily dismissed those who sought to denigrate amphetamine as a drug of abuse, stating:

> All the evidence indicates that the amphetamines are valuable and useful drugs in a wide variety of clinical conditions, and that under the circumstances of their use by millions of people, the occasional reports of habituation or untoward reaction are extremely insignificant. (Leake 1958)

During this era almost all the supplies of amphetamine came from legitimate pharmaceutical companies who overproduced the drug and appeared to turn a blind eye to diversion of supplies. Amphetamine in the USA production increased from 3.5 billion doses in 1958 to more than 10 billion doses in 1970. Amphetamine itself was available under many different trade names: Benzedrine, Dexamin, Dexamyl, Dexedrine, Synatan, Appetrol. Not only did the drug manufacturers present a variety of amphetamines to choose from, they also offered them in brightly coloured tablets or capsules, from basic white to the green of Dexamyl, the orange of Dexedrine, and the rose of Benzedrine, and some were romantically heart-shaped. Long-acting capsule formulations came in multiple hues, including green and white, orange and white, and pink and white. An extensive black market developed, with an estimated 50 per cent of commercial supplies diverted into illicit channels (Sadusk 1966). In 1966, amphetamine tablets could be purchased on the black market for $1.00 per dozen. The illicit drug was widely available at truck stops, petrol stations, and restaurants. In 1964 a TV journalist set up a bogus 'import–export' company and used the company's false notepaper to obtain more than a million doses of amphetamines and barbiturates from nine drug companies (Grinspoon and Hedblom 1975). When sales became more strictly regulated in the USA, large quantities of amphetamines continued to be sent to non-existent 'drugstores' in Mexico, where they were picked up to be smuggled back into the USA. As late as 1971, Griffith *et al.* (1971) commented that: '. . . diversion of amphetamine from legitimate distribution is so efficient that illegal tablets are available in almost every American city and cost little more than if the item were to be bought through a pharmacy'.

Despite the warnings, amphetamines continued to be prescribed and used in large quantities for both medical and non-medical uses throughout the 1970s and 1980s.

Some famous amphetamine misusers

During the 1960s and 1970s, when amphetamine misuse was not viewed as being particularly dangerous, many famous artists, film stars, politicians, and other celebrities fell victim to its seductive charms. In a number of major cities a special breed of physicians, the 'Dr Feelgoods', emerged who were willing to administer shots of amphetamine as 'pick-me-ups' to their wealthy clients. Several such doctors practised in New York during that period. The most famous example was Dr Max Jacobson who practised in Manhattan during the 1960s and 1970s. His activities were exposed by the *New York Times* newspaper in December 1972. Jacobson administered injections to his clients, alleging that they contained a mixture of vitamins, but D-amphetamine also appears to have been a major ingredient. He purchased around 80 g of the drug every month— enough for 100 large doses every day. His list of patients included more than 100 people in high-ranking positions in government, journalism, finance, industry, the diplomatic corps, society, and the entertainment world. His most famous clients were President John Kennedy and his wife Jackie. Jacobson frequently visited the White House and often travelled with the Kennedy family. In 1961 he accompanied President Kennedy to Vienna where a crucial summit meeting

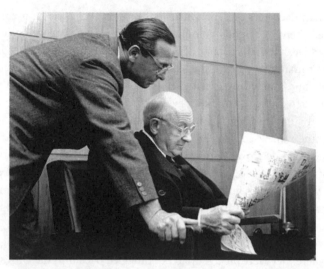

Figure 5.2 'Dr Feelgood'(Dr Max Jacobson) (standing) with one of his famous clients, the Hollywood film producer Cecil B. de Mille.

with the Russian leader Khrushchev took place. It is alleged that the President, who suffered from chronic pain and ill health, took a shot of amphetamine to prepare him for the meeting! Another famous client was the Hollywood film producer Cecil B. de Mille, who took Jacobson with him to Egypt as his guest and personal physician during the shooting of the epic *The Ten Commandments* (Fig. 5.2). Patients would go to Jacobson's office at 56 East 58th Street in Manhattan at all times of the day or night to receive their injections. Some came daily, others weekly, and some came only once a month—and received a supply of vials for self-medication. No-one could become a client other than by word of mouth from others. Jacobson did not become personally rich from his activities but seemed to relish the opportunity to mix with the rich and famous. He defended himself vigorously against the newspaper allegations, claiming that most of his patients did not receive amphetamine injections and that those that did were given only small doses. However, after an investigation that lasted more than 2 years, the New York State Board of Regents revoked his medical license in 1975.

In the entertainment world one of the tragic victims of amphetamine was the star Judy Garland (Fig. 5.3). She was already on the stage at the age of six and became a star at a very early age. Her seventh film, *The Wizard of Oz*, in which at the age of 17 she first sang her signature song *Over the Rainbow*, became an all-time classic. But the pressures of fame were high. Her Hollywood film contract required her to lose weight and she started taking Benzedrine, and then added barbiturates to counteract the insomnia caused by the amphetamine. She became dependent on these cocktails of psychotropic drugs, and her physical

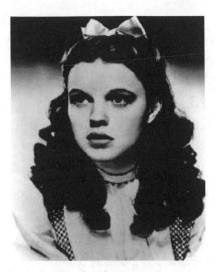

Figure 5.3 Judy Garland at the height of her fame.

and mental health deteriorated. Attempts to stop led to intolerable withdrawal symptoms and suicidal states. By 1949, at the age of 27, she began the first of many stays in a psychiatric hospital and was subjected to electroconvulsive therapy. She suffered from pain and sleeplessness and over the years her behaviour deteriorated, becoming increasingly irascible, erratic, and disruptive, and demoralizing to her remaining family and friends. Garland was a great artist and managed to summon the will for several successful comebacks, but by the 1960s she had succumbed once more to amphetamine, allegedly taking as many as 40 Ritalin (methylphenidate) tablets a day. In 1969 Judy Garland, sick both physically and mentally, largely as a result of her drug history, died from an overdose at the age of 47.

Among other famous entertainers, the singer Eddie Fisher also became addicted to amphetamines, to which he was introduced initially by Max Jacobson. Fisher describes his colourful experiences, which included a brief period of marriage to Elizabeth Taylor, in his book *Been There Done That*:

> By the time I was thirty-three years old I'd been married to America's sweetheart and America's femme fatale and both marriages had ended in scandal; I'd been one of the most popular singers in America and had given up my career for love; I had fathered two children and adopted two children and rarely saw any of them; I was addicted to methamphetamines and I couldn't sleep at night without a huge dose of Librium. And from all this I had learned one very important lesson: There were no rules for me. I could get away with anything so long as that sound came out of my throat. (Fisher and Fisher 2003)

Elvis Presley also took amphetamines. Elvis did not drink, but he abused drugs for most of his life. He is said to have began using Benzedrine to give him a lift when he began his rock-and-roll career in the first half of the 1950s. It is possible that amphetamines were first given to him by Memphis disc jockey Dewey Phillips, who helped popularize Elvis's music by playing his songs repeatedly. The drugs are said to have 'transformed the shy, mute, passive "Baby Elvis" of those years into the "Hillbilly Cat".'

In the Beat Era of the 1960s, poets and jazz musicians wove amphetamine into their subculture. Allen Ginsberg said that he wrote his classic poem *Kaddish* on a 3-day speed binge. The great jazz musician Charlie 'Bird' Parker habitually dipped an amphetamine-soaked cotton strip from a Benzedrine inhaler into his coffee. The frantic beat comedian Lenny Bruce was prescribed Benzedrine for narcolepsy, but soon acquired a dependence on the drug.

The growing menace of methamphetamine abuse in the USA
Methamphetamine was as widely available on prescription as D-amphetamine during the post-war period, marketed mainly for narcolepsy or obesity under various trade names: Methedrine, Oesoxyn, Ambar, Methampex, Desefedrin, and Desoxyn. Combination products containing methamphetamine and a sedative barbiturate (pentobarbital) were marketed as Desbutol or Obedrin.

The first US epidemic of intravenous methamphetamine abuse started in California in the 1960s and was triggered by the inappropriate prescribing of the drug for heroin dependency (Lake and Quirk 1984). This 'pseudo-medical' use spread, and some physicians were also willing to write illicit prescriptions. The most popular of the injectable ampoules were made by Abbott (Desoxyn) and Burroughs Wellcome (Methedrine). During the first half of 1962 over half a million ampoules were prescribed. One of the groups involved was the original 'Flower Power' hippie generation of drug users in the Haight-Ashbury region of San Francisco, where methamphetamine (speed) began to replace hallucinogenic drugs such as LSD in popularity.

The San Francisco Bay area became home to a large and growing number of intravenous methamphetamine users. Tolerance to the drug led to escalating use, and users became known as speed freaks (see Chapter 2). The US Department of Justice, alarmed by the rapid increase in prescriptions for intravenous methamphetamine, persuaded Abbott and Burroughs Wellcome to restrict the use of the injectable methamphetamine products to hospital patients only. This action left intravenous methamphetamine users without a product which could be injected readily. Demand was created for an inexpensive water-soluble powder form of methamphetamine, and this demand was soon met by the growth of illicit methamphetamine laboratories in California.

The growing problem of intravenous amphetamine abuse in the US during the 1960s was finally recognized by the medical community. Kramer *et al.* (1967) wrote in the influential *Journal of the American Medical Association*:

> Abuse of amphetamine administered intravenously has become a well established and extensive form of drug abuse. The abuse potential of these dugs when taken intravenously is greater than when taken orally and is comparable to that of heroin or cocaine.

To begin with the illicit manufacturers were inexperienced and the product they sold was an equal mixture of the active form D-methamphetamine with the inert isomer L-methamphetamine. The purity of the final product was also low, and fake samples containing cold remedies such as ephedrine, phenylpropanolamine, or caffeine were common. However, by the mid 1980s the average street product contained more than 70 per cent methamphetamine, and the manufacturers had learned how to synthesize the more potent single isomer D-methamphetamine. Initially, methamphetamine manufacture and sale was dominated by outlaw motor cycle gangs, in particular the Hell's Angels. Methamphetamine ('crank') was ideally suited to the biker lifestyle, which emphasized fast high-risk motor-cycling, fighting, heavy drinking, partying, and drug use (Thompson 1967). Methamphetamine manufacture and use spread to other regions of the American West Coast and eventually came to be dominated by large-scale criminal gangs from Mexico.

In a belated attempt to control amphetamine misuse, the US Government passed the Controlled Substances Act 1970, which made it illegal to possess amphetamines without a prescription. All forms of amphetamine were classified as Schedule II drugs. Partly because of these restrictions and a public information campaign 'Speed Kills', run in the early 1970s, there was a marked reduction in amphetamine use after 1972 (Miller 1997). For a couple of decades another potent psychostimulant drug, cocaine, replaced methamphetamine in popularity.

However, in another part of the USA, Hawaii, a new and highly pure form of D-methamphetamine ('ice') became available in the 1980s (Cho 1990; Laidler and Morgan 1997). Initially imported from the Far East, ice, known locally in Hawaii as 'batu' and later in mainland USA as 'crystal meth', was a clear crystalline form of methamphetamine hydrochloride resembling rock salt or candy (Fig. 5.4). It was commonly smoked or injected, and because of the high purity and the rapid absorption that smoking or injections permit it proved to be highly addictive. The native population of Hawaii had traditionally favoured locally grown high-quality cannabis (known as 'pakololo'), but government measures to crack down on cannabis use in the 1980s encouraged a switch to ice. Hardly any of the users connected ice with amphetamines; most viewed it as

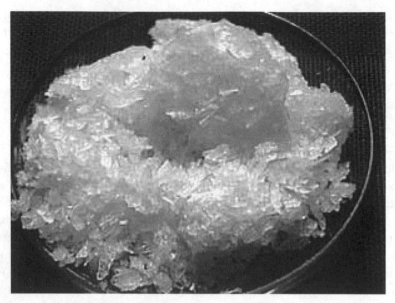

Figure 5.4 Methamphetamine hydrochloride (ice, crystal meth).

an entirely new and safe drug. Use patterns often involved prolonged binges lasting for several days, followed by the inevitable 'crash' (see Chapter 2 & Para 5.2). The epidemic that rapidly followed the introduction of methamphetamine to Hawaii had devastating disruptive effects on family and societal relationships. One man described the downward spiral of his relationships:

> Later in my addiction I started to get abusive, more abusive than ever! 'Cause of the paranoia, I couldn't handle it. My wife was trying to help me to quit but I didn't listen. The greed and my addiction got the best of me. My life with my family started to deteriorate. My son started doing his own thing 'cause he seen me doing my own thing. I was too busy to notice that my family life was falling apart. It deteriorated slowly. I wasn't paying attention to my family, I was just concentrating on my using. She would come home from work and I'd still be smoking. When she got up to get dressed for work in the morning, I'd still be up smoking . . . When she did voice opinions later, it was too late. I was too far into the addiction and making money. Twice after that she tried to get me into treatment. I never went. (Laidler and Morgan 1997)

Although methamphetamine abuse has been endemic in Hawaii for more than 20 years, the number of users seeking treatment continues to rise, and in recent years has exceeded the number presenting for treatment of alcoholism, making ice Hawaii's number one drug problem (S. Apgar, *Honolulu Star Bulletin*, 7 September 2003).

Ice soon spread to California and other West Coast states, where consumption continued to escalate. Methamphetamine is known by a number of street names: ice, speed, meth, crystal, crystal meth, chalk, and glass are common terms in the USA (Schliefer1998).

By the beginning of the twenty-first century methamphetamine abuse had become what the US DEA described as 'the most important home-grown illicit drug problem'. According to the US Department of Health and Human Services *2002 National Survey on Drug Use and Health*, more than 12 million people aged 12 and over (5.3 per cent) reported that they had used methamphetamine at least once in their lifetime (up from 8.8 million in 2000). More than half a million of those surveyed had used the drug within the previous month. Hospital emergency department visits in which methamphetamine was mentioned were up from 13 505 in 2000 to 17 696 in 2002. The US Department of Health also reported that the rates of admission for methamphetamine/amphetamine treatment rose from 10 to 52 admissions per 100 000 between 1992 and 2002. In 1992 only 12 per cent of admissions reported smoking the drug, whereas by 2002 this figure had increased to 50 per cent. Some Western states had much higher rates of treatment admission in 2002; the highest rates were 324 per 100 000 in Oregon, 217 per 100 000 in Hawaii, and 200 per 100 000 (http://oas.samsha.gov/2k5/meth/meth.htm).

The US company Quest Diagnostics, which performs more than 10 million workplace drug tests each year, has reported a rapid rise in those testing positive for methamphetamine, up from 25 per 10 000 tested in 2000 to 49 per 10 000 in 2003, with a rise of more than 40 per cent in positive tests in the year 2002–2003 alone.

Although illicit manufacture started in California, it has spread to all parts of the USA. In 2003 the DEA raided and destroyed 7050 illicit methamphetamine laboratories, of which only 709 were in California. Because methamphetamine laboratories contain so many dangerous chemicals and solvents, the DEA has trained many hundreds of special agents to undertake this work, wearing protective clothing and taking special safety precautions. The number of staff employed by the DEA increased from 2775 in 1972 to 9629 in 2003. As *Newsweek* reported in March 2004:

> The use of meth is soaring, with no end in sight. In the past year police busted more than 7000 meth labs nationally, a nearly 500 percent increase since 1996. Meth is making its way to the East Coast, but the problem 'has exploded' in the middle of the country, says Rusty Payne, a spokesman for the Drug Enforcement Administration. 'Meth is now the No. 1 drug in rural America—absolutely, positively, end of question.' In Tennessee, Missouri and Arkansas—among the states with the worst problems—meth is overwhelming law-enforcement efforts to combat the homemade drug.

Methamphetamine, traditionally the number one illicit drug for the rural poor, has now spread to major US cities. It has become the fastest growing illicit drug in the gay community in clubs and bars (Sanello 2005). The prevalence of use among gay men is twice the national average. Because of its powerful sexual stimulant effects (see Chapter 2) some gay men, sometimes using it in conjunction with Viagra, indulge in weekend-long drug and sex binges. In San Francisco, officials at the Department of Public Health estimated that up to 40 per cent of gay men in the city had tried methamphetamine. Use has spread to gay communities in other major US cities (Los Angeles, Chicago, and New York). What makes methamphetamine use especially dangerous for gay users is the correlation between methamphetamine use and HIV infection. The danger of sharing injection needles is compounded by the fact that, while on the drug, some gay men take increased risks with unsafe sex that they would not ordinarily take.

The most recent entry to the US methamphetamine scene is 'yaba'. These are brightly coloured tablets containing D-methamphetamine, often with caffeine and sometimes flavoured like candy (grape, orange, vanilla). Yaba originated in the Far East. The tablets are usually taken by mouth but can also be crushed into a powder which can be snorted or injected, or the tablets can be smoked by heating on metal foil or in a pipe. As with so many aspects of the methamphetamine story, yaba use emerged first in California, imported from the Far East by the Asian community. It has become particularly popular at rave parties, where ecstasy is also used (see Chapter 7). No doubt yaba will also spread from California to other regions of the USA.

Morgan and Beck (1997) interviewed methamphetamine users in California and Hawaii and asked them why they used the drug. The most common answers were for energy enhancement, improved performance, heightened sexuality, enhanced socialization, and improved confidence, clarity, and focus. But sadly most methamphetamine users admitted that these positive objectives were usually not achieved—the adverse consequences of drug use greatly outweighed the benefits.

5.5.2. Amphetamines in the UK

History

The first references to the misuse of amphetamines in the UK came in newspaper reports in 1937, shortly after the introduction of Benzedrine. Although the drug was freely available over the counter, one major chain of pharmacies decided to supply it only on prescription. A number of other pharmacies followed this lead, but amphetamine was still easily available. The technique of extracting large doses of amphetamine from the Benzedrine inhaler device was soon imitated in the UK. The inhalers were freely available; their sale was not even restricted to registered pharmacies. Inhaler abuse in turn led to the first examples of patients with 'amphetamine psychosis' being admitted to psychiatric hospitals (see Chapter 6). The Pharmaceutical Society was so concerned about inhaler abuse that it initiated an approach to all the manufacturers of these devices asking for their cooperation in dealing with this problem. The manufacturers responded to this appeal; some withdrew their product from the market, and others altered the formulation to include an unpalatable additive to deter improper use.

The growing use of amphetamine prompted the government to place it in Schedule 4 of the Poisons Rules current at that time, making it available from pharmacies only by doctor's prescription. However, during the 1950s its use grew as doctors wrote large numbers of prescriptions for amphetamine and its analogues as anti-obesity agents and antidepressants. The combination products that contained D-amphetamine together with a barbiturate (e.g. Drinamyl), used as dangerous and ineffective antidepressants (see Chapter 3), were particularly popular in the UK. Doctors continued to extol the medical virtues and safety of the amphetamines. A medical text published in the mid-1950s reviewed a great variety of medical indications, and the authors dismissed the possibility of addiction or abuse:

> Purposely a special section has not been included on addiction to amphetamine, as the existence of addiction is still *sub judice*. In the meantime, however, it can be stated quite categorically that addiction, using this term in its proper sense, does not occur. It is true that some psychopaths have been known to take enormous doses, but having once found the dose that suits them, unlike real addicts they have experienced no need to increase it further, and on being deprived of the drug, have shown no withdrawal symptoms. Nor is there any antisocial element in their taking of this compound. (Bett *et al.* 1955)

This is, of course, patent nonsense which flies in the face of reality. In the same year the British psychiatrist P. H. Connell published a classic monograph describing amphetamine-induced psychosis as a far more common outcome of amphetamine abuse than had previously been recognized (Connell 1958). Connell also had no doubt that his patients were addicted to the drug (see Chapter 6).

By the 1960s, as in the USA, there was widespread diversion of medical supplies of amphetamine products to illicit users. British doctors wrote 4 million amphetamine prescriptions in 1966, but equally large quantities were used illegally. The police reported widespread trafficking in D-amphetamine tablets and capsules and in the combination product Drinamyl. A newspaper article in 1970 described the teenage use of amphetamines:

> Amphetamines are the teenagers' basic drug, although most of them use several drugs and will abuse even the most homely and unlikely drugs such as Marzine travel sickness pills. The most popular pills are Drinamyl; they used to be called 'Purple Hearts' and are now known as 'French Blues'. They are a combination of amphetamine (stimulant) with a barbiturate (sedative). Amphetamine alone

often makes young takers too restless even for their own liking, but many of them still take one of the many Dexedrine-type preparations available in multi-coloured capsules or tablets—'Yellow Bellies', 'Black Bombers', and so on. (V. Brittain, *The Times*, 22 September 1970)

The popularity of amphetamines waned somewhat during the 1970s as attention focussed on heroin and cocaine, but widespread abuse continued almost unnoticed (Klee 1997a,b). During the 1980s and 1990s a new generation of young people started using amphetamine in the nightclub scenes associated with punk rock and Northern Soul. Later, it became a common drug in the rave dance scene, often combined with LSD or ecstasy.

Methamphetamine has never attained the popularity in the UK that it has in Japan or the USA. In 1968 there was a minor epidemic of methamphetamine abuse in London as a result of some doctors prescribing injectable metham-phetamine (methedrine ampoules) to cocaine addicts as a substitute. This was as misguided as the corresponding prescription of methamphetamine in California for heroin addicts. Two doctors in particular overprescribed large amounts of methamphetamine and some was diverted to the black market. The epidemic was short-lived, as in 1968 there was a voluntary agreement by the manufacturers to limit the supplies of injectable methamphetamine to hospital use only.

As in the USA, some famous figures in the UK were associated with amphet-amine abuse. Perhaps the most important, in terms of the possible influence that the drug had on the course of history, was the Conservative politician Anthony Eden. He was one of the most promising politicians of his generation. By the early age of 38 he became Foreign Secretary. By 1952, he was tipped to succeed Winston Churchill as Prime Minister.

Just when his future promised so much, a medical mishap changed the course of Eden's life for ever. During an operation to remove gallstones the surgeon damaged his bile duct. This blunder made Eden vulnerable to recurrent infections and attacks of violent pain and fever. To overcome this weakness Eden was prescribed Benzedrine, the wonder-drug of the 1950s. At that time amphet-amines were used in a very casual way; a fellow politician admits to taking them to help him deliver a tricky speech at the Conservative Party Conference. However, Eden's use of amphetamines was potentially more worrying. When, in 1955, he at last became Prime Minister, he still suffered from being in the shadow of the great war leader Churchill. To combat this insecurity and boost his confi-dence Eden began to dose himself with more and more Benzedrine. But what Eden did not know was that over time amphetamine users acquire tolerance and tend to increase their doses, exposing themselves to irritability, mood swings, perceptual changes, and paranoia. By the summer of 1956 Eden was a man with serious health problems who was regularly taking a mind-altering drug.

In July 1956 Eden faced a major international problem. Egypt's leader, Colonel Nasser, announced the nationalization of the Suez Canal Company which had been run by the UK and France since its construction in 1869. The Suez Canal was the main route that brought Middle Eastern oil to Europe, and so the UK saw the protection of its interests as vital. Eden wanted to reverse the nationalization, but he also displayed a paranoid personal animosity towards Colonel Nasser that showed all the hallmarks of a man in the grip of amphetamines. On 16 October 1956 Eden agreed to collude with France and Israel in an underhand operation. The Israelis were to invade Egypt, so that the UK and France could intervene as peacekeepers and re-occupy the Canal Zone. In former times Eden would never have considered this subterfuge, but by now he was, in his own words, 'practically living on Benzedrine'. This massive blunder led to a nuclear confrontation between the superpowers, and the UK had to undertake a humiliating withdrawal of its forces. Eden's handling of Suez had proved a disaster. But his next move surprised everyone—he went on holiday. With British troops still on the ground in Egypt, Eden's doctors sent him to Jamaica to try and break his reliance on amphetamines. This rest cure did nothing to save Eden's career. Who knows whether without the combination of illness and amphetamines Eden could have gone on to be as a good a Prime Minister as he had been Foreign Secretary. Sadly, however, he is remembered for his mistakes and for the shame of Suez.

In the British entertainment world the Rolling Stones, the epitome of the swinging sixties, were often in court for drug offences. In 1967 Mick Jagger was convicted of the illegal possession of four amphetamine tablets, which he claimed were prescribed by his doctor 'to stay awake and work'. He was sentenced to 3 months imprisonment, but this was later quashed on appeal. The Beatles were also no strangers to the 1960s drug scene. Their first exposure to illicit drugs was allegedly amphetamine from a Benzedrine inhaler given to them by an English version of Allen Ginsberg—Royston Ellis, known as the 'beat poet'.

Amphetamine abuse in the UK today

The most recent surveys of the population in England and Wales indicate that amphetamines are the fifth most commonly used drugs, after cannabis, cocaine, ecstasy, and amyl nitrate (Condon and Smith 2003). Approximately half a million people admitted to having used amphetamines during the previous year (the surveys do not distinguish between amphetamine and methamphetamine). Nearly a third of 20–24-year-olds admitted to having used amphetamine at least once in their lifetime.

What sorts of people take amphetamines? Klee (1997b) undertook a series of detailed studies of drug-users' lifestyles in Northwest England in the period 1990–1995. She had many categories, including 'controlled and uncontrolled users', 'recreational users', and 'self-medicators'. Although these data are now somewhat dated, they give an interesting picture of the various groups to whom amphetamines appeal. Some examples are given below.

Ravers

A raver is a useful shorthand term to describe a person who goes out, usually with friends, on a Friday or Saturday night to dance more or less continuously until dawn. Rave dancers have a number of different music styles, and their own magazines and commercial radio programmes. They are mostly under 25 years of age and are strictly weekend users of amphetamine; two or three friends often share a gram of amphetamine. The purity of street amphetamine is low (about 5–10 per cent), and so the dose is typically quite weak. Most will take amphetamine orally, dabbing it on the tongue or swallowing it. They tend to dislike combining amphetamine with alcohol, but will take it with LSD or ecstasy. Ravers say that amphetamine helps them to overcome anxiety and socialize more easily in a friendly atmosphere; another important factor is the energy needed for continuous dancing for several hours.

Amphetamine is widely used at dance parties and clubs in the UK; many ravers regard it as an essential and harmless part of their main leisure pursuit, and it is a cheap night out.

Speeding drinkers

This is an entirely different group. They are mainly young men who are part of drinking groups who regularly go out 'pubbing' with their friends at weekends. They find that amphetamine is a useful way of avoiding drunkenness during long drinking bouts. It gives the insecure or those who cannot 'take their beer' confidence and allows them to keep up with their friends. Many of these young men binge drink for most of the weekend. They like the confidence and composure that amphetamine gives them—not risking letting friends down through incapacity due to drink.

Young mums

These are women who had children while in their teens and are now in their mid-twenties. Their friendships are often limited to other mothers, with whom they share child-minding. They may or may not have a male partner, or their partner may be unemployed or working only sporadically. They are 'self-med-icators'; their main aim in taking amphetamines is to have enough energy to look after their children and home, and still have some free time for leisure. They will go out to clubs or pubs with women friends and use amphetamine to lift their mood and energy levels. The drug is nearly always taken orally, in drinks, dabbed, swallowed, or sometimes snorted. Higher doses may be used to undertake some major household task (decorating or cleaning). The drug has another bonus; it helps them to avoid becoming obese. There is a wide range of use, from low doses (perhaps half a gram once a week) to regular use of a gram or more a day several times a week.

The attraction of amphetamine for these women is that they believe that it meets many of their needs and helps them to enjoy what would otherwise be a claustrophobic and tedious lifestyle. They are still young and interested in dancing and socializing and an opportunity to forget their domestic chores and responsibilities.

The prudent user

These are people who use amphetamine occasionally, usually in low dose, and always for a particular purpose, such as playing football, decorating, house cleaning, driving for a long distance, going to an all-night party, or even staying up to watch television. Some will use it at work for a particular purpose. There has to be some value associated with using the drug; it is not driven by hedonism.

Prudent users are often highly informed. They are very aware of the consequences of excess and the dangers of addiction, and the pros and cons of various routes of administration:

> I'm not saying I'm sensible, because no-one is sensible if they're taking drugs, but I do try to cut the risks. I'll say I'll do this because if I don't, this'll happen. If you're snorting it it's burning a hole in your nose for a kick off and if you're injecting it isn't . . . But if you're injecting rubbish it's going to do you damage as well' (Dave, 25 years)

This group has a cautious approach to life in general. They dislike excess because it means lack of control. It is unlikely that they will become problem users.

Criminal users

Both men and women sometimes use amphetamine to boost their confidence and alertness when committing petty crime. Women prefer shop-lifting, while men tend to be responsible for burglary and theft from cars. The men often belong to groups whose activities are focused on communal drug use and crime. They are particularly common in deprived public-sector housing estates where unemployment levels are high and prospects are poor. Amphetamine is regarded as a functional aid by these groups; it keeps them awake and alert at night and gives them confidence, and they can run faster if pursued.

Conclusions from the UK experience

Although the illicit use of amphetamines is common in the UK, it does not represent the social problem seen in Japan or more recently with the methamphetamine epidemic in the USA. There appear to be substantial numbers of regular amphetamine users; according to the UN International Narcotics Control Board (United Nations 2005) the UK has the highest rate of amphetamine use in Europe. Amphetamines are the second most common illicit drug seized in the UK (after cannabis). Relatively few users appear to be severely dependent on the drug; speed freaks are relatively unknown. A survey of regular drug users indicated that the majority of those who used amphetamines regularly were 'invisible' to the police or drug services; they expressed little or no concern about their drug use, and no wish for help or advice (Robson and Bruce 1997). Nevertheless, users, particularly those who inject intravenously, risk harm. A survey in Edinburgh (Peters *et al.* 1997) revealed that amphetamines were injected by more subjects (44 per cent of their sample of injecting drug users) than any other drug. The hazardous practice of needle sharing is just as common among amphetamine users as in those who use heroin (Klee 1997b) and the risk of infection with HIV/AIDS or hepatitis is real.

The relatively low harm ratio in UK amphetamine users may be partly because methamphetamine has not been widely available or used. The majority of users take amphetamine sulphate and on the whole they take it orally. As discussed previously there are reasons to believe that amphetamine is a less addictive drug than methamphetamine, and it is well established that the oral route is less likely to lead to addiction than injecting or smoking the drug.

However, there is no room for complacency. Methamphetamine abuse may spread to the UK in the same way that it spread in the past few years from the West Coast to the East Coast in the USA. Amphetamine abuse has not so far received a high priority for punishment or treatment in the UK. As one commentator put it:

> In the sometimes sensational world of illicit drug reportage, there is one unsung villain. While heroin misuse remains the *bête noir* of tabloid journalism, ecstasy the demon of the dance floors and cocaine caricatured as the choice of the rich and famous, amphetamine misuse has lurked in the shadows. Its use defies such simple categorisation and spans several groups in society. (Cantwell 2000)

The special case of khat

Chewing the fresh leaves of the khat shrub is a habit that is endemic in certain regions of East Africa and the Arab Pensinsula where the shrub grows. Khat has an effect similar to the psychostimulant actions of amphetamines. It causes some users to become more alert and talkative; khat chewing sessions are usually highly social occasions and have an important role in the culture of these communities, where alcohol is forbidden. The active ingredient in the plant is cathinone (Fig. 2.3), which is very similar chemically and pharmacologically to D-amphetamine. Studies of the pharmacology and behavioural actions of cathinone have confirmed that it acts like D-amphetamine to release dopamine in the brain, and also possesses sympathomimetic properties peripherally (Kalix 1992). Furthermore, in drug discrimination experiments experimental animals or human subjects were unable to distinguish cathinone from D-amphetamine (Kalix 1992). The two drugs have similar potencies.

Cathinone is unstable chemically and khat loses its taste and potency after 3–4 days. However, with air freight it has become possible to provide fresh supplies of khat to those permitted to use it anywhere in the world. The UK has substantial immigrant Somali, Yemeni, and Ethiopian communities, many of whom indulge in khat-chewing, taking advantage of the fact that until now the UK government has not controlled the plant product under the Misuse of Drugs Act 1971 (although the chemical cathinone and the related substance cathine are controlled substances). Khat chewing appears to do relatively little harm in the immigrant communities, although it can sometimes lead to psychotic reactions and possibly to domestic violence. There is little evidence that dependence or tolerance develop. However, khat is a controlled product in many other European countries and in the USA. There is concern that the UK may have become a distribution centre for the import of fresh khat (mainly from Mombasa, Kenya) for illegal export elsewhere. Customs authorities estimate that as much as 10 tonnes of khat enters the country every week, far more than could be consumed by the immigrant groups in the UK.

5.5.3. Methamphetamine in Japan

The post-war epidemic of methamphetamine abuse in Japan serves as a frightening example of how easily the drug can take over the lives of millions of people when it is freely available with no health warnings (Hemmi 1969; Suwaki 1991; Fukui *et al.* 1994; Konuma 1994). From 1942 onwards methamphetamine was widely used by the Japanese armed forces to enhance wakefulness and performance. The government also encouraged its use, sometimes by coercion, by civilian workers in the industries supplying the war effort to boost their productivity. At the end of the war several factors combined to create the conditions for a very rapid growth in methamphetamine use. The Japanese population faced social confusion, poverty, unemployment, and a shortage of food and housing on an unprecedented scale. Life was hard and defeat hard to bear; the national mood was depressed. At the same time pharmaceutical companies who had supplied the war effort were left with large supplies of methamphetamine. The drug was freely available over the counter, under the trade names Hiropon and Sedorin, and the companies launched an advertising campaign with the slogan 'Fight sleepiness and enhance vitality'. This slogan had an immediate appeal to the many people who had used the drug during the war, and who were suffering from depression and a loss of confidence in the future. They were eager to experience the euphoric and mood-elevating effects of the drug. At the same time large military stocks of the drug were dumped onto the illegal market. Use of the drug spread rapidly to nightworkers, students, artists, writers, bartenders, and waitresses, and later to all walks of life. By the autumn of 1946 doctors were already beginning to see chronic methamphetamine addicts, and the first attempt to control the use of methamphetamine was made in the Drug Control Law of 1948. But the drug was still too easily available and its use continued to spread rapidly in both cities and rural areas. Groups of young people stayed out all night and abused the drug for pleasure. By 1948 it was estimated that 5 per cent of all those in the age group 16–25 years were using methamphetamine. Many users switched from the tablet form of the drug to injectable methamphetamine, taken intravenously, known generically as Wake-amine or Philopon. The imposition of much stricter controls in the Stimulants Control Law in 1951, limiting the availability of the legal drug, failed to stop the epidemic. With restrictions on the legal sources of supply, illicit manufacture and imports met the increasing demand, often with products of very poor quality which sometimes contained only caffeine or other substitutes.

At its peak in 1954 more than half a million people in Japan from all walks of life were abusing methamphetamine, mainly by intravenous injection. During the period 1945–1954 some 2 million people had used the drug in one form or another. Addicts using the injectable drug were regularly taking as much as 30–180 mg a day, and this led to the first large-scale occurrence of 'amphetamine psychosis', with large numbers of patients entering psychiatric hospitals with schizophrenia-like symptoms (see Chapter 6). In 1954 the Stimulant Control Law was further strengthened, imposing penal sanctions on illegal use of the drug, and in this year there were more than 50 000 arrests. In 1958 the law was tightened still further to control the availability of precursor chemicals and to widen the penalties for illicit production. Finally, the epidemic subsided as punishments were strictly applied and addicts were forced to enter treatment programmes. Public sentiment was also influenced by widely publicized homicides committed by methamphetamine addicts. For example, in 1954 a youth with a history of methamphetamine abuse murdered a 10-year-old girl while under the influence of the drug, triggering widespread public outrage (the Kyoko incident). By 1957 and during the following decade there were less than 1000 arrests annually under the Stimulant Control Law.

However, the methamphetamine problem had not gone away, and after 1970 abuse of the drug again spread rapidly throughout Japan. This second wave of methamphetamine abuse started initially among organized criminal gangs known as 'yakuza' and people within their sphere of influence. The drug was smuggled into the country and sold by the criminal syndicates to finance their activities. Methamphetamine abuse started with those in contact with the criminal gangs—in the construction industry, restaurants, bars, cabaret and gambling establishments, and in real estate—but soon spread more widely. Initially, many people took the drug to stay awake at night, to enhance their concentration, and to relieve fatigue. However, people were soon using the drug primarily to obtain its euphoriant effects (Fukui *et al*. 1994; Konuma 1994). A further strengthening of the penalties available under the Stimulant Control Law of 1973 had only a minor impact on the growth of methamphetamine abuse. By 1976 the number of arrests had again risen above 10 000 annually, and continued to rise rapidly to 22 000 in 1981. By then it was estimated than there was a total of 300 000 methamphetamine users in Japan. As in the previous epidemic, hospital admissions with the symptoms of 'amphetamine psychosis' once again rose to more than 3000 annually (Fukui *et al*. 1994).

Konuma (1994) gave a detailed classification of patterns of methamphetamine abuse in Japan which serves as a valuable aid to understanding the various ways in which the illicit drug is used. The same patterns almost certainly apply universally. He described six categories of methamphetamine use.

1. *Occasional use* The frequency of methamphetamine use in this group is irregular, usually once or twice a month. They may inject the drug a couple of times in the course of a night-long mah-jongg or gambling session. Occasionally they may purchase a packet of drug from a dealer and inject the drug two or three times a day until the supply is used up.

2. *Regular use* The lives of many regular users are not disrupted by their use of methamphetamine and they can continue normal work. A barmaid may inject a single dose of the drug every evening before going to work, or a truck driver may take one or two injections to stay awake during long-distance journeys on a 2-day shift.

3. *Cyclic used* Cyclic users repeat a pattern of frequent injections over a short period of time, followed by a drowsy period ('crash'). The users inject high doses (30–60 mg) two to six times daily for several days. This pattern is the same as that of the 'speed binges' first seen in California in the 1960s.

4. *Daily high-dose use* Some cyclic users shift to a daily high-dose schedule (300–500 mg in four or five doses) but manage to maintain a 5–6 hours sleep pattern and consume food as usual, avoiding the 'crash'. However, this is a fragile equilibrium and such users usually suffer a 'crash' as soon as they abstain from the drug.

5. *Compulsive use* Cyclic users may become compulsive users if they suddenly gain access to a substantial amount of methamphetamine. They use the drug compulsively at high doses (300–1000 mg per day), injecting 8–10 times daily for as long as 10 days, or until the supply is used up. This often results in a toxic psychosis and hospital admission, inevitably followed by a 'crash'.

6. *Single high-dose use* A typical single high-dose user injects 300–1000 mg in a single -injection. This habit is sometimes seen in methamphetamine addicts who resume the habit after abstinence.

Konuma (1994) noted that users often switch between these categories, influenced by a number of different factors, with a major one being how much methamphetamine they can afford to obtain. Cyclic users also develop tolerance to the drug, which may explain why they sometimes resort to single high-dose use.

The growth of methamphetamine abuse in Japan during the 1970s led to an increase not only in psychiatric hospital admissions, but also in violent crimes committed by methamphetamine users under the influence of the drug. The Fukagawa incident in June 1981, when two housewives and two infants were murdered by a methamphetamine user in Fukagawa, Tokyo, raised a storm of public protest. There was also a rapid growth in the criminal underworld responsible for supplying the drug. Methamphetamine abuse had become a serious social problem. The Japanese government further tightened the law and exerted a stricter enforcement of the Stimulant Control Law. The number of arrests peaked at 24 372 in 1984 and then decreased to 15 267 in 1990.

However, the criminal yakuza gangs had grown rich on the profits of their drug dealing, and they continue up to the present day to control illicit drug dealing by their organization of illicit import routes and widely dispersed distribution networks. Methamphetamine remains the most widely used illicit drug in Japan. Every year there are 15 000–25 000 arrests and an estimated 1–2 million users. Because of tight controls on the availability of precursor chemicals, almost all of the estimated 20 tonnes of methamphetamine used in Japan every year is imported illegally from China, Taiwan, the Philippines, and in recent years North Korea. As much as a third of the methamphetamine used in Japan originates from North Korea, which has made trade in this and other illicit drugs into a major export earner, worth as much as $500–$1000 million annually. The cost of street methamphetamine, known as 'shabu', has gone down significantly in recent years; a typical dose of 30 mg could be bought for around $17 in Tokyo in 2003.

> A typical pattern of recruitment of new users is typified by Hitoshi, who was only 16 when he came across his neighbour shooting up. It wasn't a shock—the neighbour was a member of the yakuza, and Hitoshi himself had already begun inhaling paint thinners. 'You shouldn't keep using those thinners' the neighbour told him. 'Why don't you try this? Give me your hand'. With a few seconds, the rush of methamphetamine was coursing through Hitoshi's body. 'I felt so good, as if my entire hair was standing up' he recalls, spreading his fingers and running his hands up the side of his head to demonstrate. 'I got this pulse of good feeling.' Hitoshi initially obtained the drug free from the neighbour, who claimed to be acting out of 'a sense of neighbourhood', but Hitoshi soon ended up buying the drug and it was not difficult. 'It's very easy to get meth, as easy as buying cigarettes.' (*The Age*, Sydney, 24 May 2003)

Methamphetamine abuse remains a major problem in Japan. More than 90 per cent of all drug-related arrests concern methamphetamine. Because most users inject the drug intravenously, and there are no legal supplies of clean needles and syringes, a large proportion of intravenous drug users are already carriers of hepatitis C, and there is an increasing spread of the viral diseases hepatitis B and HIV–AIDS in the drug-using community. Meanwhile the yakuza grow richer and more powerful through their control of the multibillion dollar trade in methamphetamine.

5.5.4. The methamphetamine epidemic in Southeast Asia

For many years China, Indonesia, Malaysia, and the Philippines have been centres for methamphetamine production and export to satisfy the huge demand from Japan, but the abuse of methamphetamine has more recently become widespread locally within several countries in the region. Table 5.1 indicates that Asia now accounts for more than half of all the amphetamine users in the world, with some 18 million people involved (reviewed by Choury and Meissonnier 2004). Virtually all the abuse involves methamphetamine, manufactured in numerous small and large scale illicit laboratories, using precursor chemicals obtained mainly from China.

Thailand has suffered a particularly rapid and severe epidemic of methamphetamine abuse. The drug was available initially as a medical product (methedrine), known colloquially as 'ya-khayan' (diligence pill). Off-label use was common among long-distance truck drivers and other occupational groups, but abuse led to strict government controls. Illicit manufacture followed and an illegal trade grew; the drug was renamed 'ya-ma' (horse pill)

Table 5.1 Annual prevalence estimates of consumption of amphetamines (2002–2003)

Region	Number of users (million)	Percentage of population aged 15–64 years using amphetamines
Oceania	1.94	2.78
Europe	2.37	0.44
West Europe	1.79	0.58
East Europe	0.59	0.25
Americas	4.96	0.89
North America	3.46	1.25
South America	1.50	0.54
Africa	2.13	0.44
Asia	18.16	0.76
Global	29.56	0.73

Source: UN World Drug Report 2004. [www.unodc.org/pdf/WDR_2004/Chap2_amphetamine.pdf]

after the horse's head logo stamped on each illicit pill. By the mid-1990s methamphetamine was rebranded again to 'ya-ba' (mad/crazy pill), referring to its tendency to cause psychosis in heavy users. By then it was estimated that there were more than 250 000 people with methamphetamine dependence in the country. While production was initially based locally, in recent years a flood of illicit methamphetamine has entered Thailand from the neighbouring Yunnan Province in China, and from the Shan province of eastern Myanmar (Burma). This comes in the form of ya-ba tablets that can be taken orally or crushed and injected or smoked. In a cruel marketing ploy many of the tablets are fruit flavoured and sweet, appealing to ever younger users, in a manner similar to the marketing of sugary alcoholic drinks ('Alcopops') by the Western drinks industry. It was estimated that a billion ya-ba tablets entered Thailand from Myanmar in 2003. Youngsters swallow ya-ba tablets after school and clamour for more. It costs less than a bottle of beer and the effects last for up to 10 hours. Thai teenagers view ya-ba as a cheap local form of ecstasy that lets them dance the night away. They see it as a harmless party drug.

This growth in supply led to a dramatic increase in the numbers of methamphetamine users in Thailand (Gearing 1999; Choury and Meissonnier 2004). As many as 50 per cent of the population in northern villages adjacent to the Myanmar border use ya-ba, and nationwide in Thailand the number of methamphetamine abusers rose by more than 10-fold in less than a decade. With an estimated total of 2.5 million methamphetamine abusers (more than 5 per cent of the population), in 2001 Thailand had the highest prevalence of methamphetamine abuse in the world. The Thai government seems to have had little success in addressing the very serious social problems that this led to. The initial reaction was the launch of military attacks by the Thai army against territories in southern Myanmar held by the Wa people, using troops and helicopter gunships in an attempt to destroy illicit methamphetamine laboratories and seize their drugs. However, this had little success in the difficult mountainous territory of Shan province and against the formidable firepower of the United Wa State Army (UWSA). In 2003 the Thai government launched a ferocious attack on drug traffickers and users in its own country, resulting in the deaths of thousands of people in an action that gained much international criticism for violation of human rights. This too seemed to have only a small effect in limiting the methamphetamine epidemic. Meanwhile the Wa drug traffickers continued to bribe an increasing number of senior Thai government officials and members of the Thai armed forces to turn a blind eye to their trade. The current Thai government appears to have given up on direct military action against the Myanmar drug manufacturers, but seems intent instead on a policy of détente with the Myanmar government, hoping that by promoting peace and prosperity that country may be weaned away from the drug trade (T. Fawthrop, *Asia Times Online Co Ltd*, 2003).

Thailand is not the only country in the region suffering from dramatic increases in methamphetamine abuse. The Drug Enforcement Agency in the Philippines estimated that there were 3.4 million drug users there in 2003, most using methamphetamine ('shabu'). Apart from local illicit drug manufacturing groups, the Philippines also serves as a staging post for Chinese drug barons exporting to Japan and to other neighbouring countries. In 2003 police seized more than $100 million worth of drugs and laboratory equipment (T. Cerojano, *Manila Bulletin*, 12 July 2003, www.mb.com.ph 2003).

In Cambodia, which shares a border with Thailand, methamphetamine abuse has reached epidemic proportions. Until only a few years ago the US DEA regarded Cambodia as 'the only Southeast Asian country without a significant drug abuse problem'. However, since 2000 there has been a sudden influx of ya ba from neighbouring Thailand, and a large increase in the numbers of dependent methamphetamine abusers. In a country in which 60 per cent of the population are under the age of 25, and the majority work long hours in the subsistence farming economy, it is not hard to see why the drug has such appeal, boosting energy, stamina and euphoria. A teenage boy, Sony, described his experience on a small Cambodian farm as follows:

> At his farm in remote Phnom Proek district, a former Khmer Rouge stronghold on the Thai–Cambodia border, Sony says, all the male workers smoked the drug they call by its Thai names of 'yaba'. He first tried it at age 12, when friends took turns waving a lighter under tablets on foil or in bottles and then sucked the milky smoke into their lungs through a straw. Yet others swallowed the purple or orange tablets whole so the effects would be milder but last longer. A few had already picked up the new fashion from Thailand of mixing it with their blood and injecting it into each other's veins with a shared syringe.

The drug also appeals to the middle-class disco-hopping youth of Cambodia. Some estimates indicate that 50 per cent of all young people in Cambodia have tried methamphetamine at least once, and the number of regular drug abusers is growing more rapidly there than in any other Asian country (www.cambodi-anonline.net/articles2004119.htm).

China is not immune from the methamphetamine problem. It has already become a major player in terms of the supply of the precursor chemicals needed for illicit manufacture and increasingly in the local production of the drug. In March 2005 a Chinese drug baron, Liu Zhaohua, was arrested in his home town of Fuan City, accused of the illicit manufacture in northwest China of up to 14 tonnes of methamphetamine with a street value of more than $5 billion (*Shanghai Morning Times*, 8 March 2005). If convicted he will face the death penalty.

There seems no end in sight to the current Southeast Asian methamphetamine epidemic, which continues to spread. Until some control can be gained over the flood of illicit supplies of the drug there seems little hope of containing the further recruitment of large numbers of dependent users in this region of the world.

5.5.5 Sources of illicit amphetamines

The first ever United Nations global survey on ecstasy and amphetamines was reported in September 2003 (United Nations 2003). It revealed a striking picture of increase in production and trafficking of these drugs. Over the past decade seizures of amphetamines have risen 10-fold to almost 40 tonnes in 2000–2001. Estimated worldwide production is more than 500 tonnes a year. A large part of the increase in the use of amphetamines occurred in East and Southeast Asia where the illicit manufacture and consumption of methamphetamine has increased dramatically in the recent past. This region of the world accounted for two-thirds of all amphetamine seizures in 2000–2001 (United Nations 2003).

Methamphetamine use has also increased rapidly in the USA, and in most European countries D-amphetamine remains the most common stimulant for non-medical use.

There is no longer any significant diversion of legitimate medical supplies of amphetamines to illicit channels, but the drugs are still freely available. One of the problems in attempting to control the abuse of amphetamines is that they are very simple chemicals which can be manufactured fairly easily in quite large quantities even by amateur chemists operating illicit laboratories. These range from individuals preparing the drugs in small amounts in their kitchens to large-scale factories operating in Mexico and in the remote jungles of the Far East or Latin America. In particular, they provide drugs to fuel the current epidemic of methamphetamine abuse in many parts of the world. Detailed instructions can be seen on numerous web sites and there are even books available to instruct the amateur chemist; the laboratory equipment needed is also readily available. Methamphetamine is a particularly popular drug of abuse in the western states of the USA, and illicit manufacturing operations have proliferated particularly in California and other western states. Some idea of this 'cottage industry' is given by the following.

> Bernard is not some Johnny-come-lately cook with a jailhouse recipe in his jeans. He is a second-generation outlaw who at 16 learned how to extract pure methamphetamine from common industrial chemical solutions in a laboratory hidden on an Indian reservation. He was tutored by two German chemists flown in by his father. Bernard can't pronounce methylamphetamine, but he knows how to make something very like it and how much to charge. 'I've worked hard for everything I have,' Bernard says, proudly citing the enduring American ethic.
>
> Bernard's skills are much in demand these days. Crank sales in the revitalized industry pushed past the $3 billion mark last year. And because the 25-ton annual

demand exceeds manufacturing capacity, there has been a scramble to increase production. Here in the heartland of the meth outlaws, a territory beginning roughly at the southerly edges of the great Los Angeles metropolitan sprawl, anarchy has replaced the discipline of a monopoly maintained for decades under the mailed fist of the renegade motorcycle clubs. Southern California, a nose ahead of Texas, remains the manufacturing capital of the country, with scores, if not hundreds, of clandestine operations scattered south from Orange County to San Diego and eastward into the Mojave Desert. 'The absolute lock the bikers held has been broken, and it's now a wide-open game, with every player for himself', says Larry Bruce, a lean, bearded Orange County criminal lawyer and former public defender celebrated by the biker fraternity for his courtroom skills. (Jonathan Beaty, *Time*, April 1989)

And

Methamphetamine use is especially prevalent in western states. Meth-related hospital admissions rose 366 per cent over 10 years in California. Arizona's Maricopa County, which includes Phoenix, reports methamphetamine-linked crimes have jumped almost 400 per cent in three years. And the drug is spreading rapidly across the US. In recent months, officials have seized huge shipments of methamphetamine originating in Mississippi and Tennessee.

Meth has always been the poor man's cocaine. Like coke, it can be smoked, snorted or injected, but 'it's much cheaper and it gives people a longer high', notes Ed Mayer, head of the Jackson County, Oregon, Narcotics Enforcement Team. For decades, its manufacture and distribution was a low-level enterprise dominated by motorcycle gangs. The current surge is driven by powerful Mexican syndicates, which have found that meth offers far greater profit margins than cocaine or heroin.

Meth does not require huge, heavily guarded growing fields or sophisticated equipment. It can be cooked up by amateurs with a few simple chemicals in makeshift labs hidden away in cheap motels, mobile homes or isolated farms and ranches. Just $4000 in raw ingredients converts to 8 lbs of meth worth $50 000 wholesale.

Speed kitchens flourish in California because the Mexican syndicates smuggle ephedrine, a key ingredient that is tightly controlled in the US, across the border. In 1994 authorities busted 419 clandestine labs in California, compared with 272 in all the other states combined. 'What Colombia is to cocaine, California is to methamphetamine', says Bill Mitchell, special agent in charge of the DEA's San Francisco office. (Anastasia Toufexis, *Time*, 8 January 1996)

Since those articles were written illicit methamphetamine laboratories have continued to spread to many other parts of the USA, particularly in the mid-West. However, the small amateur laboratories account for only a small part of the world's consumption of amphetamines. In 2002 the United Nations identified 17 countries as sources of illicit methamphetamine and amphetamine manufacture. The main source countries were Myanmar (formerly Burma), China, the Philippines, North Korea, and Mexico (United Nations 2003).

In Europe, the Netherlands has become a centre for D-amphetamine production, perhaps because of its easy access to world trade routes to source the precursor chemicals needed. Countries in Eastern Europe have also traditionally also been centres for the manufacture of illicit amphetamine and methamphetamine, and more recently the rave-dance-culture drug ecstasy. The historic role of Czech Republic was explained by a spokesman for the Czech National Anti-Drugs Centre in January 2003 as follows:

> . . . already during the communist period, with almost completely restricted state borders, there was a relatively strong industrial base formed for illicit drug production, from small chemical laboratories to well-equipped shops for the manufacture of methamphetamine, better-known in the Czech Republic as Pervitin.
>
> This fact indeed was the reason Pervitin became known as 'the Czech drug'. Pervitin was first made in Japan in 1888. In 1943, in the Protectorate of Bohemia and Moravia, the Third Reich Patent Management patented the manufacturing process of Pervitin. Production factories were built by Herman Goering in northern Bohemia, and Pervitin itself, due to its strong psychotropic and stimulating effect, was delivered to Japanese kamikaze pilots and to special brigades of the SS and Wermacht.
>
> Simply for historical reasons, there was no other place in the world where Pervitin was made in such quantities and with such a well-organized industrial base.

Much of the illegally manufactured methamphetamine uses the drug ephedrine as starting material (Fig. 5.5), although this is not the only route of manufacture. Ephedrine is a natural product made by the *Ephedra* shrub and it has mild amphetamine-like properties. It was used in Chinese medicine as a stimulant more than 5000 years ago and has been known to Western medicine for many centuries. Ephedrine is legally available in many parts of the world, although bulk supplies are now illegal in the USA and Europe because of the diversion to illegal methamphetamine manufacture. However, ephedrine in capsule form is still freely available as a medicine. It is used as a nasal decongestant, appetite suppressant, and mild stimulant to enhance performance. Ephedrine is made from natural sources and can also be chemically synthesized.

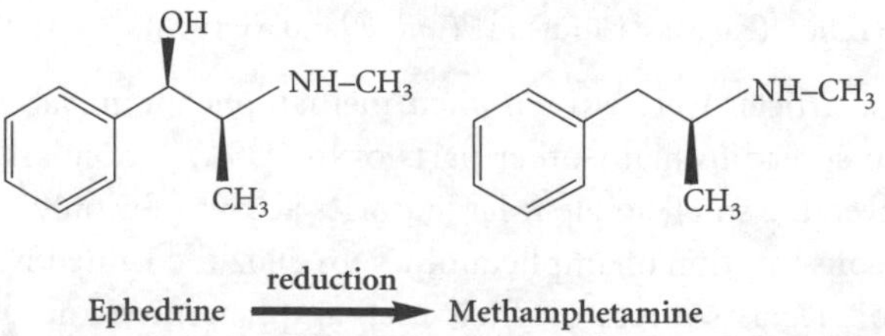

Figure 5.5 The natural herbal medicine ephedrine can be converted chemically to methamphetamine.

The use of ephedrine as a starting material yields methamphetamine of high purity in the more active D-isomer form. Pseudo-ephedrine is also widely available as an ingredient in cough/cold medicines and it can also be used a starting material to produce D-methamphetamine. A powerful reduction step is needed to convert ephedrine or pseudo-ephedrine to methamphetamine. There are various ways of achieving this, but they all involve very reactive and hazardous chemicals: sodium or lithium in liquid ammonia, or red phosphorus and iodine. Highly inflammable solvents are also used. Another compound of herbal origin, norephedrine (which lacks the *N*-methyl substituent of ephedrine), can also be used as a starting material with similar chemistry for the synthesis of D-amphetamine.

Illicit methamphetamine manufacturers also use a different chemical route employing phenylacetone, methylamine, and formic acid as starting materials (Fig. 5.6). If hydroxylamine is used instead of methylamine, this provides a way of manufacturing amphetamine. Again, there are several alternative routes of synthesis, but they all involve toxic and hazardous chemicals. When phenylacetone is the starting material it yields a less pure product containing a mixture of the D- and L-isomers and a variety of contaminants, often including toxic heavy metals, such as lead, which are used as catalysts. Most of the illicitly manufactured amphetamines are of very poor quality, often with as little as 10 per cent purity.

Given the nature of the materials used it is not surprising that the illicit producers and their families frequently suffer from poisoning or laboratory accidents and fires. Scott (2003) gives a graphic account of the hazards experienced by those who operate illicit methamphetamine laboratories, their children, neighbours, and family members, and the law enforcement and other personnel who have to enter such places. Methamphetamine production is often carried out in unsuitable poorly ventilated locations such as hotel rooms where a build-up of toxic fumes can occur and the risk of explosion is increased. Premises in which methamphetamine production has taken place will often be found to be widely contaminated with methamphetamine and various noxious chemicals. A further unfortunate consequence of this industry is that for every

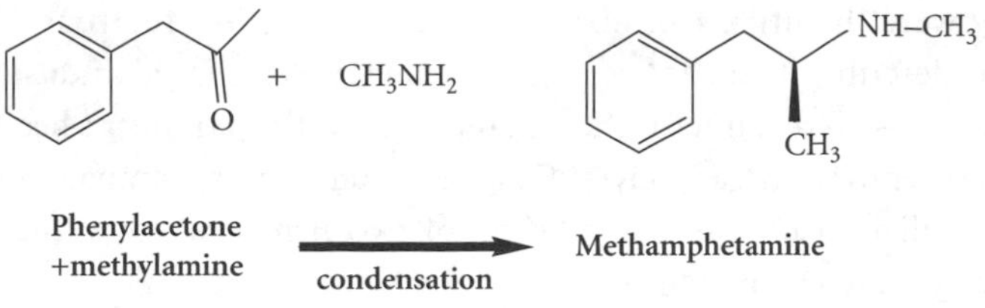

$$\text{Phenylacetone} + \text{CH}_3\text{NH}_2 \xrightarrow{\text{condensation}} \text{Methamphetamine}$$

Phenylacetone
+methylamine → condensation → Methamphetamine

Figure 5.6 Alternative route for synthesis of methamphetamine widely used in illicit laboratories.

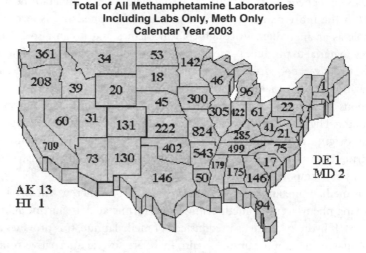

Figure 5.7 Illegal methamphetamine laboratories closed in the USA in 2003.

kilogram of methamphetamine produced there are several kilograms of highly toxic chemical waste and solvents, which are usually dumped indiscriminately to contaminate ground and water supplies.

In 2003 more than 7000 illicit methamphetamine laboratories were seized, mainly in the USA (Figs 5.7 and 5.8). Clandestine operators are increasingly using the Internet to find out where laboratories can be set up most favourably, how to access precursor chemicals, and how to find corrupt officials to bribe. The business is estimated to have an annual value of $65 billion, with profit margins as high as 3000–4000 per cent. Given these tempting returns and the ability to set up manufacture with relatively simple equipment, it is unlikely that this industry will be easy to shut down.

In Southeast Asia the illicit manufacture of methamphetamine, in the form of ya ba, is dominated by the Wa people in the remote mountainous southern region of Myanmar. This fiercely independent group resisted the advances of the British Empire. In 1893 a British colonial administrator named George Scott launched the first expedition into wild Wa territory. He demolished the myth that they were 'habitual cannibals' with a predilection for roasted babies. Instead he described them as '. . . an exceedingly well-behaved, industrious and estimable race—were it not for the one foible of cutting stranger's heads off and neglecting ever to wash themselves'. Despite brutal military campaigns by Scott's men, in retaliation for the decapitation of two British officers, the Wa were never brought under colonial rule.

The Wa had traditionally grown the opium poppy and traded in opium, and during the latter half of the twentieth century they developed a flourishing

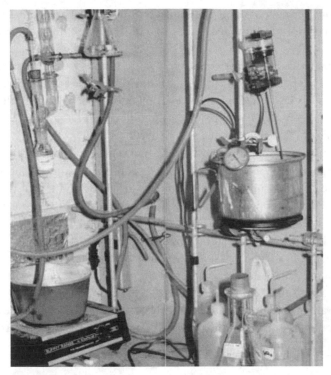

Figure 5.8 Part of an illegal methamphetamine laboratory in California.

export trade of opium and heroin to Thailand. The drug trade came to be dominated by the UWSA, a formidable force of tribal soldiers described by the US State Department as the world's 'most heavily armed narco-traffickers'. This is a truly remarkable force, with some 20 000 soldiers, heavily armed with the latest military technology including heavy machine guns, artillery, anti-tank weapons, and Chinese-built shoulder-fired surface-to-air missiles (A. Marshall and A. Davis, *Time Asia*, 16 December 2002). Every Wa family with three or more children must send conscripts for training in the army. The UWSA maintains strict discipline and there are harsh punishments for any soldiers caught using ya-ba. They control the border with Thailand and an export industry valued at more than $500 million annually. The Wa-based drug industry is thought to have plans to expand its operations into nearby Laos and the Yunnan province of China, thus gaining the possibility of access to new markets in China and India. Shipments of ya-ba are already turning up in Europe, Australia, and the USA. The attitude of the military junta who govern Myanmar and the Wa tribal leaders to the UWSA appears equivocal. On the one hand, they publicly deplore the narcotics traffic; on the other, they seem to welcome the strong military presence of the UWSA on the country's southern border.

Money-laundering has meant that funds from Wa groups have found their way into the control of many businesses, including a bank, in other regions of Myanmar, and no doubt in the form of bribes to helpful government officials. Wa leaders proclaim themselves determined to stamp out the narcotics trade, but all that has been done so far is a commitment to eradicate the opium/heroin trade. This has involved the forcible eviction of tribal peoples from the mountain slopes where the opium poppy has traditionally been grown. These mass relocations of Wa people have caused great suffering to those displaced, and to the unfortunate people into whose already poor villages a host of forced immigrants has been dumped. A total of 100 000 people may ultimately be displaced by the end of 2005, and any farmers who try to stay behind to cultivate opium poppies will be stopped by what are described as 'executive measures'. The relocations seem to have had little effect on the opium trade so far, but the Wa can claim to be doing something about the drug trade, while continuing to expand their business in ya-ba—a drug that is far easier to export and is not subject to the vagaries of the weather or spy satellite surveillance (A. Marshall and A. Davis, *Time Asia*, 16 December 2002). The Wa drug baron Wei Hsueh Kang is wanted in both Thailand and the USA for drug trafficking. The US State Department has put a $2 million reward on his head (T. Fawthrop, *Asia Times Online Co Ltd*, 2003).

CHAPTER 6

Amphetamine psychosis: how research on amphetamines provided new insights into the brain mechanisms underlying schizophrenia

6.1. History

Almost as soon as Benzedrine was introduced as a medicine, there were reports of adverse psychiatric reactions to the drug. The first description of a drug-induced psychosis was given by Young and Scoville (1938) who described a state of paranoid psychosis in two patients who were being treated for narcolepsy with Benzedrine. However, these authors suggested that the reaction was probably due to the presence of some degree of psychiatric abnormality prior to Benzedrine treatment and recommended that patients be screened for such symptoms before drug treatment. Herman and Nagler (1954) also described psychotic reactions in eight patients who had been regular Benzedrine abusers, chewing the contents of Benzedrine inhalers to obtain 250–500 mg of the drug daily. The typical reaction resembled a paranoid psychosis with auditory and visual hallucinations together with agitation and excitement. Herman and Nagler also seemed to attribute these reactions to the patients' previous history which they said 'uniformly revealed evidence of social maladjustment and psychopathy'.

During the period leading up to the Second World War and in the 'honeymoon' period for more than decade after the war amphetamine became increasingly widely used for a variety of medical indications and Western medicine generally considered it to be safe. Between 1945 and 1958 there were only 17 reports of amphetamine-induced psychosis in the USA (and only nine cases of amphetamine dependence) (Kalant 1973).

However, on the other side of the world in Japan the post-war period saw the world's first major epidemic of amphetamine abuse, involving at its peak as many as a million people (see Chapter 5). Methamphetamine had been widely used by both the military and civilians during the war and large stocks were freely available in the post-war period. The drug was commonly injected intra-venously at high doses, with an average daily dose approaching 100 mg (Angrist and Sudilovsky 1978). Toxic reactions to high doses of the drug were common, and frequently involved acute psychiatric reactions. Tatetsu (1964) described 492 such cases and reported a wide range of symptomatology, including schizophrenic state, manic depressive illness, delirium, and anxiety. Perhaps differences in diagnostic criteria at that time may have explained why Western medicine subsequently described the adverse psychiatric effects of amphetamine largely in terms of paranoid psychosis. In any event, the Japanese experience showed that adverse psychiatric reactions induced by the drug were not as rare as had previously been thought, although the Japanese findings went largely unnoticed in the West for many years.

In the UK interest in the topic was stimulated by the monograph published by the psychiatrist P. H. Connell of the Maudsley Hospital entitled *Amphetamine Psychosis* (Connell 1958). In what is now regarded as a classic landmark study in the field, Connell reviewed the literature and reported on his own case series of 42 patients. He described the symptoms as clearly resembling those of paranoid schizophrenia and noted that they normally disappeared within a week of stopping the drug. Connell's clear description and his belief that amphetamine psychosis was far more common than usually assumed at the time were important advances.

In California the first epidemic of methamphetamine abuse, associated with the Haight-Ashbury 'Flower Power' generation in the 1960s (see Chapter 5) also made it clear that amphetamine-induced psychosis was a fairly common consequence of amphetamine addiction and abuse. The current wave of increasing methamphetamine abuse in the USA is bringing this unwanted reaction into focus once again.

The resemblance between amphetamine-induced psychosis and some forms of schizophrenia generated much interest in the research community. New lines of research sought to examine how close the parallels were and to probe their underlying neurochemical and neuropharmacological bases. This work was of great importance in supporting the 'dopamine hypothesis' of schizophrenia and providing insight into the mechanism of action of the anti-psychotic drugs used to treat schizophrenia as dopamine antagonists.

6.2. What is amphetamine psychosis?

As with many other aspects of human responses to amphetamines, there is a wide spectrum of individual variation in the adverse psychiatric responses induced by amphetamine. Angrist (1994) describes the syndrome most commonly seen by clinicians as

> ... a paranoid or paranoid-hallucinatory psychosis in a setting of clear consciousness in which formal aspects of thought are relatively intact but in which delusion and hallucinations frequently invoke intense fear.

He presents two case histories to illustrate these points.

> An 18-year old who had taken amphetamine orally for a year hitchhiked to New York and took 100 mg orally before going to a nightclub. There he argued with a man and left. On the street he became preoccupied with the idea that the person with whom he had argued might have called friends to 'get' him. Thus, anyone on the street might have been sent after him. He went into a bar where people seemed to be looking at him in a sinister, amused way. He left the bar and on the street was particularly frightened by people with 'flat' faces (since the person with whom he had argued originally had a 'flat' face). He went to his hotel and barricaded the door with a bed. Soon he heard a radio being played in the hall, and assumed it was being played loudly to drown out his screams as he was being murdered. He crawled out on the window ledge (on the third storey) and, while out on the ledge, heard voices saying 'Let's get him now!' At this point he decided that he had to run and ran out of the hotel with an open penknife in his had. He met a policeman while still holding the knife and asked to be taken to a psychiatric hospital. Entering the hospital, he felt he was being pursued by a large crowd of people. His symptoms cleared completely in 3 days.

The second case history described an 18-year-old man admitted to Angrist's research ward in New York.

> In the 2 weeks prior to admission he stayed in his brother's and sister-in-law's apartment and had taken 3–7 injections per day of a powder of unknown purity that he was told was methamphetamine. During this time he heard his brother tell his sister-in-law that he had killed his mother and planned to kill him (the patient) as well. He panicked, and in an attempt to escape, ran into the street without shoes or shirt and jumped on the rear fender of a passing mail truck. This led to his being taken to Bellevue Psychiatric Hospital by the police. In the hospital he was frightened, apprehensive and felt that the staff and other patients were implying that 'he knew something' that he refused to tell. When he was seen by the research staff, two days after admission (a Monday), his affect was blunt, constricted, and at times incongruent. After being transferred to the research ward he became frightened and tearful fearing that this was a place where patients were sent to be punished and perhaps even killed. He showed a formal thought disorder: on the day of his transfer, speaking of his brother's drug use he said 'My brother has been playing with the fires of hell.' ... On the next day persecutory ideation had diminished and was replaced by diffuse referentiality—i.e. other patients on the ward were looking at him

peculiarly. He was apprehensive about a female patient on the ward that he referred to idiosyncratically as 'the girl I call Bonnie' (after the movie *Bonnie and Clyde*). These mental status features then cleared rapidly (after 5 days in hospital).

Although amphetamine psychosis bears some striking resemblances to paranoid schizophrenia, there are also some important differences (Snyder 1972). Amphetamine psychosis is frequently associated with auditory hallucinations which resemble those experienced by patients with schizophrenia, including hearing vague noises and voices, and occasionally having conversations with the voices. However, amphetamine psychosis is also commonly associated with visual hallucinations, often involving faces, and visual hallucinations are rare in schizophrenia. Another form of tactile hallucination, sometimes known as 'formication', is unique to amphetamine psychosis. The syndrome begins with a sensation of tingling or itching which leads to scratching and rubbing. As delusions form, the patients may become convinced that ants, small animals, worms, lice, or crystals of amphetamine have been placed under their skin. Olfactory hallucinations may also occur. Another difference between the drug-induced psychosis and schizophrenia is that, whereas schizophrenic patients have blunted or inappropriate emotional responses, amphetamine psychosis is often associated with extreme anxiety and fear reactions. The drug taker seems to retain some insight into his state and there are clear, if delusional, thought processes; again, neither of these is characteristic of schizophrenia.

6.3. Experimental induction of amphetamine psychosis in normal subjects

The idea of deliberately inducing a schizophrenia-like psychosis in normal subjects by giving them amphetamine would probably not be considered ethically acceptable nowadays, but things were different 30–40 years ago and several such studies were conducted, although for ethical reasons they were restricted to subjects who had previously abused high doses of amphetamine.

Griffith *et al.* (1968) showed that amphetamine psychosis could reliably be induced in such 'normal' subjects. The volunteers, all with previous experience of high doses of amphetamine, received 5–10 mg of D-amphetamine by mouth every hour for as long as they could tolerate it. All four subjects developed paranoid delusions, but without hallucinations or formal thought disorder. Nevertheless, since the subjects had been screened for the absence of schizophrenic symptoms at the start of the study, the results definitively answered the question of whether amphetamine could induce *de novo* psychosis or whether it merely released 'latent' schizophrenic symptoms.

Angrist and Gershon (1970) used a similar protocol but gave larger doses of oral DL-amphetamine (up to 50 mg/h). Their subjects developed paranoid delusions, and olfactory, auditory, and visual hallucinations were reported by some subjects, suggesting that the absence of hallucinations in the study by Griffith *et al.* (1968) may have been due to the use of lower drug doses. After 465 mg DL-amphetamine over a period of 23 hours, one subject experienced an acute and florid paranoid hallucinatory psychosis. He saw 'coloured halos' around lights, and then 'heard' a gang coming into the ward to kill him. He assumed that the experimenter had 'set up the trap'. He had visual hallucinations of gangsters, doors opening and closing in the shadows, and visual illusions, i.e. the paper on a bulletin board 'turning into a gangster in a white raincoat'. He jumped at the slightest sound, assuming it was the gang coming to 'get' him, and he was certain that the endpoint of the experiment was for him to be killed. Some subjects in the study by Angrist and Gershon (1970) also developed formal thought disorder after very high doses of amphetamine. After receiving a total of 595 mg DL-amphetamine, one subject became disorganized, rambling, and very bizarre. He felt that had become 'a prophet' who was being addressed directly by God. He stated:

> My consciousness in the form of what you know as human. My feeling which I received from him. I bring the answer to unknown and yet. They who do not hear or show laugh or murder my love. In my human form he might let me act human for the rest must still wonder at my actions which make them doubt my having been used to enlighten. Every thought that stops me from accepting all knowledge more than man has ever known. It is just part of the supreme game to make you wait until it is time for you to receive everlasting good. It is not mine to give. I am his. I bring his will, call it prophet.

In another study, Bell (1973) found that psychosis was produced by intravenous methamphetamine in 12 of 14 patients who had previously been addicted to amphetamine. The doses needed to precipitate psychosis varied widely, as did the duration of the effect which was 1–2 days in nine cases, 6 days in two patients, and 26 days in one patient. The two patients who did not respond were the only ones who had not previously used high doses of amphetamine. Although Bell described all his subjects as having 'seriously disturbed personalities', he did not believe that amphetamine was revealing latent psychotic traits.

The results of this research, albeit in subjects who could not be considered entirely normal as they were all previous amphetamine users, convincingly showed the power of amphetamine to induce bizarre and frightening schizophrenia-like symptoms in people who had not previously exhibited symptoms of psychosis.

6.4 Role of sensitization in amphetamine psychosis

For obvious reasons it is impossible to model amphetamine-induced psychosis in animals. However, animals exposed to repeat doses of amphetamine consistently show enhanced responsiveness to the drug, although the neurochemical mechanisms underlying this sensitization remain unclear (see Chapter 2) (Segal and Kuczenski 1996). There have been few controlled studies of amphetamine sensitization in human subjects, although many believe that this phenomenon may play a key role in determining the onset of amphetamine psychosis on repeat exposure to the drug. In a double-blind placebo-controlled study of repeated D-amphetamine challenges involving 11 healthy control subjects, Strakowski *et al.* (1996) showed that with only two doses separated by 24 hours it was possible to show enhanced drug-induced responses after the second dose. They measured activity/energy level, mood, rate and amount of speech, and eye blink rates for 5 hours after drug administration; all four parameters showed sensitization.

Ellinwood (1967, 1972) stressed that amphetamine psychosis is a gradually developing process in most regular users. Progressively more abnormal behaviours develop; feelings of being watched evolve into paranoid delusions; visual hallucinations start with fleeting glimpses of just recognizable images in the peripheral vision, and later they become fully formed and stable; auditory hallucinations begin with hearing simple noises. Kramer (1972) also described a typical pattern of progressively increased vulnerability to psychosis that develops over months of amphetamine use.

> The paranoia does not usually start during the first few months of high-dose intravenous use. When it does finally begin, it is mild, easily controlled, and is largely dissipated upon waking after crashing; and it usually doesn't start again until after two or three days on a new run. As time goes on, it may start earlier in a run and may persist to some extent even after crashing. In some instances the first injection after a period of sleep will bring about a return of the paranoia. Once an individual has experienced amphetamine paranoia, it will rather readily return even after a prolonged period of abstinence.

This all suggests that sensitization may play an important role, particularly in amphetamine-induced psychosis associated with a chronic high-dose 'binge' pattern of amphetamine or methamphetamine abuse. However, Segal *et al.* (2003) pointed out that because of the relatively slow elimination of amphetamine/methamphetamine from the body, the pattern of evolving psychosis during a single 'run' might also simply be linked to the progressive cumulative rise in blood levels of the drug during repeated dosing. However, this could not explain the progressive evolution of amphetamine psychosis over a period of months described by Ellinwood (1972) and Kramer (1972), which suggests a role for sensitization.

6.5. Relevance of amphetamine psychosis to understanding schizophrenia

6.5.1. Anti-schizophrenic drugs act as dopamine antagonists

The true madness of schizophrenia is a complex illness which is difficult to understand. Schizophrenia affects about 1 per cent of the population. It develops after puberty in early adult life, and is often a lifelong illness. The symptoms are varied and bizarre; no two patients will be quite the same. Key symptoms include auditory hallucinations (often hearing voices talking about the patient in the third person), irrational delusions, feelings of persecution and paranoia, inability to express appropriate emotions, incoherent thought processes and language, withdrawal from social contacts, and immobility. The illness often leaves the sufferer incapable of normal work or other daily activities, and the delusions may lead him or her to irrational and dangerous acts of violence towards others.

The discovery of drugs that tackle some of these key symptoms was a major advance in the treatment of schizophrenia. The first breakthrough was an accidental discovery. In the early 1950s, two French physicians J. Delay and P. Deniker, noted the remarkable calming effects of a new drug, chlorpromazine, that was initially tested as an agent used to relax patients before major surgery (Delay et al. 1952). They tested the drug in patients suffering from mania and found it to be remarkably effective. This led to tests in schizophrenic patients, where again chlorpromazine had remarkable effects in calming agitated patients without putting them to sleep; it was a tranquillizer, not simply a crude sedative. Chlorpromazine rapidly came into widespread use on both sides of the Atlantic as a new and effective treatment for schizophrenia. Many other effective anti-schizophrenia agents followed chlorpromazine, including several far more potent drugs (e.g. haloperidol, fluphenazine, and flupenthixol). Some of these drugs were up to a thousand times more potent than chlorpromazine, making it possible to deliver enough drug to last for several weeks in a single dose, usually by means of a 'depot injection' into a muscle. In this way it has proved possible to treat schizophrenia in outpatient clinics, in which medication is administered once or twice a month. The availability of such treatments was one of the factors that led to the gradual disappearance of the Victorian mental hospitals, in which patients with schizophrenia were formerly locked away.

Discovering how anti-schizophrenic drugs act in the brain has been one of the major achievements of the new subject of psychopharmacology, and two of the pioneers in this field, Arvid Carlsson in Sweden and Paul Greengard in the USA, were awarded the Nobel Prize for Physiology and Medicine in 2000. They helped to show that the key target for all the effective drugs in this class is the monoamine neurotransmitter dopamine. The drugs used to treat schizophrenia, although they come from many different chemical classes, all act to block the actions of dopamine at its receptors in the brain. It took a long time for this to become clear. Chlorpromazine and many of the other anti-schizophrenic drugs that followed it were discovered before dopamine was known to be a neurotransmitter in its own right in the brain. Previously it had been thought to be present merely as a precursor for the biosynthesis of norepinephrine. In 1958, Arvid Carlsson discovered that dopamine was present in some brain regions without norepinephrine, and probably acted as a neurotransmitter in its own right. Carlsson and Lindqvist (1963) provided the first clue about the role of dopamine in mediating the actions of chlorpromazine and related anti-psychotic drugs. They found that modest doses of chlorpromazine and haloperidol caused increases in levels of the dopamine metabolite methoxytyramine in mouse brain. They reasoned that this might be the consequence of an increased rate of dopamine release and subsequent metabolism, perhaps to compensate for a drug-induced blockade of the normal actions of dopamine in the brain. This somewhat complex reasoning turned out to be correct. More elaborate experiments to measure the rates of dopamine synthesis in rat brain confirmed that anti-psychotic drugs did indeed selectively increase dopamine synthesis and metabolism (Sedvall 1975). Sedvall *et al.* (1975) also showed that schizophrenic patients treated with anti-psychotic drugs had elevated levels of the dopamine metabolite homovanillic acid in their cerebrospinal fluid. The final demonstration of the mode of action of anti-psychotic drugs awaited the discovery of biochemical methods to study dopamine receptors. An initial phase of research concentrated on a dopamine receptor that was linked to the formation of the messenger molecular cyclic AMP discovered in Greengard's laboratory (Kebabian *et al.* 1972). This receptor (now known as dopamine D_1) was potently inhibited by anti-psychotic drugs of the chlorpromazine class (phenothiazines) and related thioxanthenes (e.g. flupenthixol), but haloperidol and related drugs of the butyrophenone class were not as potent as might have been expected from their high clinical potencies (Clement-Cormier *et al.* 1974; Miller *et al.* 1974). It was not until a second dopamine receptor (dopamine D_2) was discovered, which inhibited cyclic AMP formation, that the true target was found. Snyder's group in Baltimore studied the ability of anti-psychotic drugs to compete for the binding of a radiotracer to D_2 receptors in a test-tube system, and found a remarkable correlation between the drug potencies measured in this way and their known clinical potencies for treating schizophrenia, which had been determined previously by trial and error (Fig. 6.1) (Creese *et al.* 1976a,b). Similar findings were reported independently by Seeman in Canada (Seeman *et al.* 1975, 1978).

Amphetamine also played an important role in this developing story. In developing new anti-schizophrenic drugs, the brilliant drug discoverer Paul Janssen in Belgium found empirically that certain animal behavioural tests

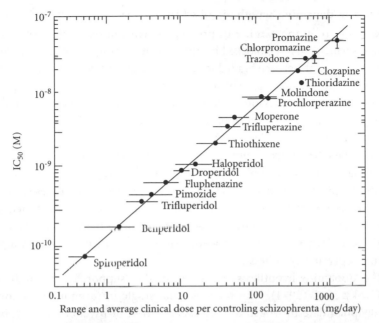

Figure 6.1 Correlation of clinical potencies of anti-schizophrenic drugs (daily dose) with *in vitro* potencies in a test-tube radioligand binding assay of dopamine D_2 receptor potencies. (Reproduced from I. Creese *et al.*, *Science*, **194**, 546, 1976.)

could be used to predict novel anti-schizophrenic drugs (Janssen *et al.* 1965). Among the most reliable tests was the ability to block the stimulant actions of amphetamine in animals, particularly blockade of the repetitive stereotyped behaviour elicited by high doses of amphetamine. Stereotyped behaviour could also be elicited by the morphine analogue apomorphine, and this also turned out to be a predictive test. Later, it became apparent that apomorphine acted directly on dopamine D_2 receptors in brain. It also became clear that the actions of amphetamine could be attributed to its ability to cause a release of dopamine in the brain (see Chapter 2). For example, the Danish pharmacologist Axel Randrup showed that amphetamine-induced stereotypies could be replicated by injection of dopamine into the dopamine-rich basal ganglia of rat brain, and that anti-psychotic drugs were 'specific antagonists of amphetamine stereotypy' (Randrup and Munkvad 1970). Randrup prophetically noted that '... knowledge about the mechanism of action of amphetamines might further the understanding of the pathogenesis of schizophrenia and the action of anti-psychotic drugs'.

Consistent with these animal data was the finding that amphetamine-induced psychosis in human volunteers could also be antagonized by anti-schizophrenic drugs (Angrist *et al.* 1974).

6.5.2. The 'dopamine hypothesis' of schizophrenia

The ability of amphetamine to provoke a schizophrenia-like psychosis in humans which could be blocked by anti-psychotic drugs provided compelling evidence for a link between brain dopamine and schizophrenic illness, and offered further support for the mode of actions of the drugs as dopamine antagonists. Although, as noted previously, amphetamine psychosis does not completely model the symptoms of schizophrenia, it comes closer than any other drug-induced psychosis (Snyder 1972). Amphetamine psychosis mirrors some of the so-called 'first-rank' symptoms of schizophrenia, and indeed many people suffering from amphetamine-induced psychosis have been misdiagnosed as schizophrenic. In the early 1970s some scientists suggested that these emerging discoveries implied that the underlying abnormality in brain function in schizophrenia might be an over-activity of dopamine mechanisms. Matthysse (1973) and Snyder et al. (1974) reviewed the evidence then available in support of the 'dopamine hypothesis'.

The 'dopamine hypothesis' was given further support by the findings of Janowsky et al. (1974), who reported that single intravenous injections of methylphenidate provoked a brief exacerbation of psychotic symptoms in schizophrenic patients. This involved modest doses of the drug, which did not provoke psychotic reactions in normal subjects. Angrist et al. (1980a) followed this up with a more elaborate series of studies involving the administration of single oral doses of D-amphetamine to schizophrenic subjects. They confirmed that amphetamine made the patients' psychotic symptoms worse, and found that those patients who responded most severely to amphetamine were also more likely to obtain the greatest benefit from treatment with anti-psychotic drugs. At about this time Tim Crow, in the UK, proposed the seminal idea that schizophrenic illness was really composed of two distinct syndromes (Crow 1980):

• the type I syndrome, consisting of florid 'positive' symptoms, which was sensitive to anti-psychotic drugs and associated with dopaminergic mechanisms

• the type II syndrome, consisting of 'negative' symptoms, such as blunted emotional responsiveness, immobility, and poverty of speech, which was not responsive to anti-psychotic drugs and was associated with intellectual impairment and possible structural brain abnormalities.

Angrist et al. (1980b) reanalyzed their findings in terms of 'positive' and 'negative' symptom scores. They found a clear distinction: only the 'positive' symptoms were made worse by D-amphetamine, and these were the symptoms which responded most clearly to anti-psychotic drug treatment. This refined the 'dopamine hypothesis' as the probable underlying cause of the florid positive symptoms of psychosis in schizophrenia, while leaving other aspects of the illness unexplained. These were landmark studies in the field of schizophrenia research and were followed by many others. Curran *et al.* (2004), in a review of stimulant-induced psychosis, identified 54 studies of amphetamine- or methylphenidate-induced psychosis in schizophrenic patients. This review showed that by no means all schizophrenic patients responded adversely to amphetamine; overall 50–70 per cent of those with pre-existing acute psychotic symptoms showed a brief exacerbation of psychosis ratings, although many patients showed no such response.Indeed, in some patients amphetamine actually improved psychosis ratings (Van Kammen *et al.* 1982). Van Kammen and Bunney (1982) reported that patients who showed the greatest amphetamine-induced worsening in their symptoms were those most likely to benefit from subsequent treatment with the anti-psychotic drug pimozide. Van Kammen *et al.* (1982) suggested that dopamine over-responsiveness is not a permanent feature of schizophrenia but is a state-dependent phenomenon, most likely to be seen in patients undergoing a florid active stage of the illness and less likely to occur during periods of stable illness.

The emergence of the 'dopamine hypothesis' prompted several laboratories to seek direct evidence for abnormalities in the dopamine system in the brains of schizophrenic patients. Early studies concentrated on measurements of neurotransmitters and their receptors in samples of brain tissue obtained post-mortem. Several studies did indeed find elevated levels of dopamine (Bird *et al.* 1979) and dopamine D_2 receptors (Lee *et al.* 1978; Owen *et al.* 1979; Cross *et al.* 1981). However, the interpretation of these findings proved equivocal because the majority of schizophrenic patients involved in such studies had received long-term treatment with anti-psychotic drugs. Mackay *et al.* (1980) and Iversen and Mackay (1981) reported elevated D_2 receptor binding sites in post-mortem brain samples from 21 drug-treated schizophrenic patients, but no such increases were seen in tissue samples from seven patients who had been drug free for a month or more prior to death. Animal studies clearly showed that chronic treatment with anti-psychotic drugs led to elevation in the density of dopamine receptors in brain, presumably as a compensatory change in response to drug-induced receptor blockade (Burt *et al.* 1977; Seeman *et al.* 1978).

Subsequent studies applied brain imaging methodology to assess brain dopamine receptors in the living human brain, using tracer doses of radioactively labelled anti-psychotic drugs that bind with high affinity to dopamine D_2 receptors. These studies were confined to schizophrenic patients who had not received anti-psychotic drug treatment to avoid any complications. However, the results were again ambiguous. Although one group reported elevated dopamine D_2 receptors in schizophrenic brain (Wong *et al.* 1997), two other studies were negative (Farde *et al.* 1990; Nordstrom *et al.* 1995). In a sophisticated variation of this approach (Abi-Dargham *et al.* 2000), brain imaging was again used but no elevation in brain dopamine D_2 receptors was found in schizophrenic patients. However, when brain dopamine was depleted by administering the synthesis inhibitor α-methyl tyrosine, a significant elevation in dopamine D_2 receptors was detected when the schizophrenic subjects were given a second radiotracer test. The authors argued that elevated levels of dopamine in the schizophrenic brain led to an increased occupancy of dopamine D_2 receptors at baseline, thus competing with the radiotracer and obscuring the true difference in receptor densities that existed. Several studies have indeed shown an increased rate of synthesis of dopamine in the brains of schizophrenic patients, as measured by an enhanced uptake of the radiolabelled precursor molecule [^{18}F]fluoro-DOPA (McGowan et al. 2004).

Most interesting from the present perspective were studies that revealed supersensitivity to the dopamine-releasing actions of amphetamine in schizophrenic patients. Three separate groups have now reported that low doses of D-amphetamine cause an increased release of dopamine in the brains of schizophrenics in comparison with control subjects. Radiotracer binding was measured by brain imaging techniques in the same subjects with and without amphetamine pretreatment, and dopamine release was assessed by virtue of its ability to compete with the radiotracer and thus reduce its binding to dopamine D_2 sites (Laruelle et al. 1996; Breier et al. 1997; Abi-Dargham 1998). Furthermore, the extent to which amphetamine-induced dopamine release was increased in individual patients correlated with the severity of their positive psychotic symptoms (Abi-Dargham et al. 1998).

Thus, although static measurements of dopaminergic mechanisms failed to reveal significant abnormalities in schizophrenia, more recent dynamic studies have been more positive. The results suggest that at least the active florid symptoms of schizophrenia may be associated with an increased synaptic release of dopamine together with a possible sensitization to the actions of dopamine (Seeman and Kapur 2000; Angrist et al. 2001; Seeman et al. 2005).

However, it is worth recalling that amphetamine does not cause a worsening of psychotic symptoms in all patients, and even in individual patients the response may depend on the stage of their illness (Van Kammen et al. 1982). Davis et al. (1991), in a review of the 'dopamine hypothesis', sought to refine it. They suggested that while the positive symptoms of schizophrenia may be related to excessive dopamine activity in mesolimbic brain areas, the negative/deficit syndrome might be related to abnormally low dopamine activity in the prefrontal cortex. In some cases boosting dopamine activity could be beneficial, if the balance between negative and positive symptoms lay towards the negative rather than the positive syndrome.

Nowadays most scientists believe that the biological basis of schizophrenia will eventually be understood in terms of an abnormality in brain development. Modern genetic approaches are already beginning to identify several possible risk factor genes, some of which are related to mechanisms known to be important in the development of brain circuits and synapses (Harrison and Owen 2003). It is interesting that only one of the risk factor genes identified to date has any connection with dopaminergic mechanisms; this is the enzyme catechol-O-methyl transferase (COMT) which plays an important role in the inactivation of dopamine in the prefrontal cortex (Harrison and Owen 2003; Mattay *et al.* 2003). However, regardless of the ultimate biological basis of the illness, the 'dopamine hypothesis' has played an important role in helping understanding of the neurochemical basis of some of the cardinal features of the illness. Although no short-term drug-induced effects can ever accurately mimic the symptoms of complex and chronic psychosis, amphetamine comes closer than any other. Research on amphetamine in animals and in human subjects has contributed importantly to these ideas.

CHAPTER 7

How dangerous are the amphetamines?

7.1. Introduction

All drugs, even such apparently innocuous ones as aspirin, carry some health risks. But how dangerous are the amphetamines? Can an overdose kill you? Does amphetamine abuse cause damage to the health and social lives of the users and those around them? Are there any long-term irreversible adverse effects of chronic use? In this chapter we will attempt to answer some of these questions and review the extensive literature on the neurotoxicity of amphetamines studied in animal experiments.

7.2. Acute toxicity

7.2.1. Effects of overdose in humans

According to the US Department of Health and Human Services *2002 National Survey on Drug Use and Health*, hospital emergency department visits in the USA in which amphetamine or methamphetamine was mentioned increased from 25 245 in 1995 to 38 961 in 2002; methamphetamine was mentioned in 17 696 visits in 2002. About one-third of these involved overdoses. According to the UK Office for National Statistics amphetamine-related deaths (other than those related to ecstasy) were recorded at rates of 30–50 per year for the period 1997–2001. Amphetamine-related deaths in the USA also occur at rates of several hundred per year.

The features of amphetamine/methamphetamine overdose may include chest pains, loss of speech, paralysis, coma, convulsions, shock, decreased urine output, and high fever (above 40°C). Emergency room treatment includes attempts to reduce body temperature since the most common cause of death is multiple organ failure resembling that resulting from heatstroke (Lan *et al.* 1998). Other causes of death are related to the sympathomimetic effects of amphetamines. Norepinephrine release in peripheral blood vessels and in the heart can lead to cardiovascular collapse secondary to ventricular fibrillation or cerebral stroke and haemorrhage caused by a drug-induced rise in blood pressure. There are other rarer causes of death, including bacterial infection caused by dirty injection needles, poisoning by heavy metals (e.g. lead) introduced as contaminants in illicitly manufactured supplies of drug, and liver failure (Jones and Simpson 1999).

Overdosing or 'over-amping' is rare among experienced amphetamine or methamphetamine users. Repeated use of the drugs leads to a high degree of tolerance, particularly to the dangerous sympathomimetic effects. Stimulant binging is characterized by the frequent intake of very large doses (often every 2 hours) over several days. Speed freaks may inject methamphetamine 8–10 times a day at high doses (a total of 0.2–1.0 g daily). Because of the long half-life of amphetamines in humans, these users obtain virtually constant or escalating blood concentrations during a binge. Such doses would be lethal to a drug-naive subject. In fact, the two most common scenarios for overdose and death occur when new users who have not developed tolerance take the same high doses that an experienced associate is capable of taking, or when an abuser takes a high dose after a period of withdrawal when tolerance has been diminished (Davidson et al. 2001).

The amphetamines are not as dangerous in overdose as some other illicit drugs of abuse. For example, the 'window' between recreational doses of heroin and those that cause death by respiratory depression is relatively small. Overdose and death are far more common with heroin than with amphetamines. The UK Office for National Statistics recorded 790 heroin-related deaths in 2002 and 591 in 2003, and several thousand heroin-related deaths occur annually in the USA.

7.2.2. Acute toxicity in animals

There is a large scientific literature on the effects of high doses of amphetamine and methamphetamine in animals, mostly rats and mice (Seiden et al. 1993; Gibbs et al. 1996; Davidson et al. 2001; Kita et al. 2003). Because amphetamines have much shorter plasma half-lives in rodents than in humans, repeated dosing is needed to simulate the sort of plasma levels of the drugs attained in human users during a binge. An acute dosage regime of four doses of 5–20 mg/kg injected subcutaneously every 2 hours in a single day is commonly used. This causes hyperthermia and occasional convulsions, and is associated with a high degree of mortality. In rats, body temperature may rise above 40°C after each injection. Reducing the hyperthermia by keeping the animals in a cold room (4°C) or using ice-baths reduces mortality, and these manoeuvres are frequently used by researchers who are interested in studying the long-term effects of exposure to the high-dose amphetamine regime (Davidson et al. 2001). The lethality of amphetamine in rodents also depends on other environmental conditions, such as stress. Chance (1946) showed that when mice were kept in separate cages, the amphetamine LD_{50} (the dose needed to kill half the animals) was eight times higher than when 10 animals shared a cage (117 mg/kg versus 14 mg/kg).

A majority of studies have used acute high-dose regimes, including studies in monkeys (Davidson *et al.* 2001; Kita *et al.* 2003). However, it can be argued that although these high doses cause reliable pathology, they are not very relevant to the effects of amphetamine/methamphetamine in human drug users. In particular, the animals have not generally had any previous drug exposure and thus lack any degree of tolerance. Therefore some researchers regard much of the literature on the neurotoxic effects of amphetamine in animal studies as more relevant to what happens in overdose in man (Davidson *et al.* 2001).

7.3. Long-term neurotoxic effects of amphetamines

7.3.1. Human studies

Animal studies (see below) have shown consistent evidence for persistent changes in neurochemical markers of dopaminergic nerves in the brain after exposure to high doses of amphetamine or methamphetamine, with some studies indicating actual nerve damage. There is also evidence that some of these drug-induced changes occur in the brains of chronic amphetamine/methamphetamine users (Nordahl *et al.* 2003). Several studies have found marked reductions in levels of the dopamine transporter (DAT) in the basal ganglia regions of brain in chronic amphetamine users (McCann *et al.* 1998c; Volkow *et al.* 2001) and in the prefrontal cortex (Sekine *et al.* 2003). DAT levels were assessed using positron emission tomography and the radiotracer [^{11}C]WIN-35428 which binds selectively to the transporter molecule. McCann *et al.* (1998c) found that reduced levels of DAT binding persisted in some subjects even after 3 years of abstinence, and suggested that this was evidence for irreversible neurotoxic damage to dopamine nerves. The most direct evidence for changes in dopaminergic mechanisms came from a post-mortem analysis of the brains of 12 chronic methamphetamine abusers who died within 24 hours of their final dose (eight from overdose, two from heart attacks, and two from gunshot wounds) (Wilson *et al.* 1996). There were large reductions in the levels of dopamine in the basal ganglia and nucleus accumbens (about half normal levels), with no changes in norepinephrine or serotonin. DAT levels were also markedly reduced in the basal ganglia and nucleus accumbens. In contrast, the dopamine biosynthetic enzyme tyrosine hydroxylase was significantly reduced only in the nucleus accumbens, and the binding of the radiotracer [^{3}H]-dihydrotetrabenazine, which binds selectively to the vesicular monoamine transporter in dopaminergic nerve endings, was not significantly altered. Wilson *et al.* (1996) argued that their findings indicate acute changes in dopamine and DAT levels in dopaminergic nerves in brain, but that these were not accompanied by actual damage to nerve endings since the vesicle marker and the biosynthetic enzyme remained largely intact. Nevertheless, Wilson *et al.* suggested that the reduced levels of dopamine in the brains of methamphetamine users may partly explain some of the symptoms of depression, anhedonia, and craving that they tend to experience after cessation of drug use. Reduced levels of DAT would be expected to reduce the behavioural effects of subsequent drug administration, contributing importantly to drug tolerance. Reduced dopamine neurotransmission in the brains of amphetamine/methamphetamine users may also be a motivational factor in seeking further drug use in partial compensation for this neurochemical deficit.

Other imaging studies have shown impairments in brain energy metabolism (glucose utilization) in various brain regions in chronic methamphetamine users (Volkow *et al.* 2001; London *et al.* 2004). The latter authors reported that methamphetamine users in early stages of abstinence had reduced energy metabolism in the anterior cingulate, insula, and amygdala regions of cortex, and the extent of these changes correlated with self-reports of depressed mood. Wang *et al.* (2004) confirmed the reductions in energy metabolism in the thalamus and basal ganglia of methamphetamine users in early stages of abstinence (less than 6 months), but they found partial recovery towards normal levels of energy metabolism after a protracted period of abstinence (12–17 months). This recovery was accompanied by improvements in the subjects' performance in neuropsychological tests of motor and memory function, suggesting that the changes may not be permanent. Whether the alterations in energy metabolism are a consequence of the impaired dopaminergic neurotransmission is not known, but is quite likely.

Thompson *et al.* (2004) used high-resolution MRI to look for signs of structural damage to the brains of 22 long-term methamphetamine users (average duration of drug use, 10.5 years; average weekly dose, 3.44 g) compared with 21 controls. They reported surprisingly large changes in the drug users' brains, with an overall increase in white matter volume (+7 per cent) and the volume of the fluid-filled brain ventricles (+19.6 per cent), indicative of a loss of grey matter. The damage appeared to be particularly severe in the hippocampus (decrease in volume of 7.8 per cent), and the extent of the hippocampal change in individual subjects correlated with the severity of deficits in tests of verbal memory. These results are impressive since, as the authors point out, the magnitude of the changes reported are as great as those seen in the early stages of Alzheimer's disease, and are suggestive of substantial drug-induced brain damage. However, it remains to be seen whether these findings can be replicated and there are some confounding features. For example, most of the methamphetamine users were also tobacco smokers, and other studies have found reduced levels of grey versus white matter in smokers, although these changes were not selective for the hippocampus (Brody *et al.* 2004). Furthermore, not all studies on amphetamine users have found deficits in memory function (Chang *et al.* 2002). It is possible that the data reported by Thompson *et al.* (2004) may not represent methamphetamine-induced changes alone.

7.3.2. Animal studies

Effects of acute high-dose amphetamine/methamphetamine treatment

The extensive literature on animal studies of amphetamine-induced neurotoxicity has been reviewed elsewhere (Seiden *et al.* 1993; Gibbs *et al.* 1996; Davidson *et al.* 2001; Cadet *et al.* 2003; Kita *et al.* 2003). Most studies used rats treated with a high-dose drug regime for one or more days. The dose used was typically 4×10 mg/kg subcutaneously at 2-hour intervals, which was sometimes escalated as animals became tolerant. A consistent finding is that dopamine levels are markedly reduced (by around 50 per cent) in most brain regions and this is accompanied by a comparable reduction in DAT. After regimes using very high doses there is also a loss of the vesicular monoamine transporter and evidence for actual damage to dopamine-containing nerve endings, evidenced by an activation of microglial cells, characteristic of nerve degeneration. However, the cell bodies of the dopamine neurons remain intact. Some rodent studies have shown that these neurochemical changes are reversible. Cass and Manning (1999) found that the evoked release of dopamine and dopamine uptake were reduced 1 week and 1 month after methamphetamine, but these functional losses were much less by 6 months and had completely recovered by 1 year. Guilarte *et al.* (2003) found evidence for two types of neurotoxicity in rat brain after methamphetamine. In the basal ganglia and central grey matter of the brainstem the loss of dopamine and DAT was accompanied by a loss of the vesicular monoamine uptake sites and by glial activation indicative of neurodegeneration, but in other regions of brain they found evidence of less severe damage, with reduced dopamine and DAT but no loss of vesicular monoamine transporter or glial activation.

However, the alterations in dopaminergic neurochemistry appear to be more permanent in primates. Seiden *et al.* (1976) found a marked reduction in dopamine levels in monkey basal ganglia which persisted for 3–6 months after drug administration. Woolverton *et al.* (1989) reported that basal ganglia dopamine levels were still reduced 4 years after drug withdrawal, but Melega *et al.* (1996, 1997) found evidence for partial recovery of dopaminergic function in vervet monkeys 6 months after amphetamine treatment, with almost complete recovery after 2 years.

Several studies have reported changes in serotonin-related neurochemical markers, with amphetamine-induced reductions in the levels of serotonin and the serotonin transporter (5HTT), but there is less evidence for drug-induced neurodegenerative damage to serotonin-containing nerve endings (Davidson *et al.* 2001; Kita *et al.* 2003).

In summary, treatment of rodents and monkeys with high doses of amphetamine or methamphetamine leads to marked changes in both dopamine and serotonin function. After the most severe dosage regimes, this may be accompanied by neurodegenerative changes suggesting a 'pruning' of the distal terminals, particularly in dopaminergic neurons. Although these changes persist for weeks or months following drug treatment, there is evidence that they may be slowly reversible as the nerve fibres gradually regenerate.

There have been many studies of the neurochemical mechanisms which underlie amphetamine/methamphetamine neurotoxicity in animals (Davidson *et al.* 2001; Cadet *et al.* 2003). Ever since the US National Institute on Drug Abuse (NIDA) was established in the 1970s it has consistently supported such basic research (Hanson *et al.* 2004). Unfortunately, almost all this research has employed very high doses of amphetamine or methamphetamine, often repeated over a period of several days. The severe damage that this causes to monoaminergic neurons does not appear to reflect accurately what occurs in chronic human amphetamine/methamphetamine users. Although there are reductions in the levels of dopamine and DAT in the brains of human users (see section 7.2.1), there is little evidence that this is accompanied by the long-term degeneration of monoaminergic nerves seen in animal experiments. Animal experiments have shown that a single exposure to a high dose of amphetamine or methamphetamine can cause rapid downregulation of DAT function, which is not accompanied by structural damage to dopamine nerves (Fleckenstein *et al.* 2000; Zahniser and Sorkin 2004). This has not stopped NIDA from warning that abuse of methamphetamine can lead to irreversible damage to the brain (Volkow 2005).

In animals, amphetamine-induced dopamine neurotoxicity is clearly related to hyperthermia. Thus keeping rats at 4°C markedly lowers the extent of reduction in dopamine levels induced by methamphetamine (4×10 mg/kg) (Bowyer *et al.* 1994). Similarly, treatment with a variety of drugs that lower body temperature also has a protective effect (Albers and Sonsalla 1995; Davidson *et al.* 2001).

In terms of the cellular mechanisms involved in amphetamine-induced neurotoxicity, most hypotheses have focused on the role of 'oxidative stress' (Davidson *et al.* 2001; Cadet *et al.* 2003). This means that there is an increased formation of reactive oxygen species (e.g. hydrogen peroxide, nitric oxide peroxynitrite),which are highly chemically reactive molecules that are known to precipitate cellular damage. This excess formation of dangerous chemicals is probably due to the drug-induced flood of dopamine release into the cytoplasm of dopaminergic nerves and the surrounding extracellular space. Within the cell, dopamine is readily oxidized both spontaneously and by means of the enzyme monoamine oxidase, forming reactive species in the process. Amphetamines may also enter mitochondria in the nerve ending to promote excess calcium release and formation of reactive species.

Are there better animal models for studying long-term neurotoxicity?
There have been several attempts to devise improved animal models for studying amphetamine/methamphetamine-induced neurotoxicity. The high doses used in many of the published studies on amphetamine/methamphetamine neurotoxicity bear little relation to human doses, even after allowing for the 'species scaling' effect which states that drug doses for rats usually need to be about 10 times higher than those for humans to achieve the same blood levels and effects. Human subjects can detect the psychostimulant effects of methamphetamine doses as low as 5 mg (approximately 0.06 mg/kg) (Hart *et al.* 2001). Methamphetamine addicts take doses that are usually in the range 20–40 mg (0.25–0.67 mg/kg). When designing experiments in laboratory animals it is also important to take account of the differences in the duration of amphetamine actions in these species compared with humans. Cho *et al.* (2001) pointed out that the plasma half-life of methamphetamine in rats was only 70 minutes compared with 12 hours in humans. This means that in order to simulate human drug levels in rats it is necessary to dose far more frequently. In addition, the acute treatment of animals with high doses of the drugs does not include an important feature of stimulant abuse in humans, which is the gradual escalation of stimulant does that often occurs prior to high-dose exposure. Segal *et al.* (2003) simulated this in a rat model by pretreating rats with gradually increasing doses of methamphetamine (0.1–4.0 mg/kg) over a period of 14 days prior to an acute methamphetamine 'binge' (4 × 6 mg/kg at 2-hour intervals). The results showed that the pretreatment phase had a profound influence on both the behavioural and the neurochemical results. In control rats not pretreated with the drug high-dose methamphetamine lead to prolonged and severe repetetive biting, gnawing, and licking (stereotyped behaviour) which continued for more than 3 hours after the last dose of drug. In contrast, animals that had been pretreated reacted differently to the high-dose regime; there was much less stereotyped behaviour but there was a prolonged period of intense running activity. There was also tolerance to the damaging hyperthermia response to the drug in the pretreated group. The neurochemical changes were also different; reductions in dopamine, DAT, and vesicular transporter markers were considerably smaller in the pretreated animals. More research using sophisticated animal models such as this is badly needed.

Another interesting approach was described by Stefanski *et al.* (1999). They trained rats to self-administer injections of methamphetamine (0.1 mg/kg intravenously) by pressing a lever. Other rats were 'yoked' to the self-administering animal in such a way that each time a self-administered dose was given these animals received passively either the same dose of methamphetamine or a saline injection. This experiment continued for 5 weeks, and after 24 hours withdrawal the rat brains were examined for evidence of neurochemical changes. Rats that had actively administered methamphetamine, but not the yoked controls, showed marked decreases in the densities of dopamine D_2 receptors in the ventral tegmental area and substantia nigra and D_1 receptors in the nucleus accumbens. After 7–30 days withdrawal these neurochemical changes reverted to normal (Stefanski *et al.* 2002). The finding that the effects of methamphetamine on the brain were different when animals actively self-administered the drug as opposed to receiving it passively (as in most previous studies of neurotoxicity) is intriguing and important.

The ultimate animal model may be to use a non-human primate, and Madden *et al.* (2005) have described a model in the rhesus monkey which involved a gradually escalating regime of methamphetamine doses from 0.1 to 0.7 mg/kg over a period of 4 weeks, followed by exposure to 0.75 mg/kg twice a day 20–23 times a month (to simulate human use). The results from this model are preliminary, but the gradual escalation of doses allowed tolerance to develop to the damaging hyperthermia response to the drug and the model holds considerable promise.

7.4. Adverse effects of amphetamines on human behaviour

7.4.1. Neurocognitive impairment

There is a substantial literature on the question of whether the chronic abuse of amphetamines leads to long-term impairment in cognitive function (Nordahl *et al.* 2003). This is a difficult question to disentangle, since acute administration of these drugs can enhance some aspects of cognitive function (see Chapter 3). However, there have been several reports of impaired cognitive function in long-term amphetamine users. Simon *et al.* (2000) compared 65 current methamphetamine users with 65 control non-users, using a battery of cognitive tests, and found significant deficits in verbal and visual memory tasks. McKetin and Mattick (1997, 1998) also reported deficits in verbal and visual memory tasks in methamphetamine users, but found that these were associated with heavy users and those rated to have a high level of amphetamine dependency, and were not found in low-dependence lighter drug users. Salo *et al.* (2002) evaluated attentional performance in chronic methamphetamine users who had abstained from drug use for 8–16 weeks. There were significant impairments in the drug users on various attention-based response measures, with the methamphetamine group displaying longer reaction times. The authors concluded that methamphetamine users had an impaired ability to focus attention ands to manage distraction. In a further study Simon *et al.* (2004) found that a range of cognitive impairments persisted in methamphetamine users for at least 3 months during a period of withdrawal and abstinence. Paulus *et al.* (2002) found that when 10 methamphetamine users were compared with 10 controls the drug users performed worse on simple two-choice prediction or response tasks as a measure of decision-taking ability. Brain imaging with functional MRI also showed less brain activity in the drug subjects in regions of the brain normally activated by decision-making. Some of these deficits may recover gradually during a period of abstinence. Simon *et al.* (2000) found that methamphetamine users recovered the ability to ignore irrelevant information and to manipulate information after 3 months of abstinence, although deficits in handling verbal material persisted for 5–6 months of abstinence.

However, the evidence for persistent cognitive deficits in amphetamine users and ex-users is not entirely consistent. At least one study reported normal verbal memory performance in chronic methamphetamine users compared with controls (Chang *et al.* 2002). There are problems with interpreting much of this literature. Chronic amphetamine/methamphetamine users suffer from a variety of physical and psychological problems, including general poor health, anxiety, and depression, which may interfere with their performance at the time of testing.

7.4.2. Self-injurious behaviour

In animals, high-dose amphetamine/methamphetamine treatment leads to intense stereotyped behaviour—repetitive biting, gnawing, licking, and rearing, and compulsive grooming. If the dose is high enough or repeated often enough this can advance to self-injurious behaviour, including gnawing and biting of the animal's own limbs (Kita *et al.* 2003). Self-injurious behaviours are also sometimes seen in human amphetamine users; these include self-biting, head banging, scratching, cutting, hair pulling, and other forms of tissue damage. Chronic amphetamine/methamphetamine users may develop sores and skin abscesses on their bodies from repeated scratching at 'crank bugs' in response to the common delusion that bugs are crawling under the skin. There are also instances of patients who severely and repeatedly mutilated their own genitalia while intoxicated on amphetamines (Israel and Lee 2002). Kratofil *et al.* (1996) suggested that the observation of bizarre self-injurious behaviour should alert the physician to the possibility of amphetamine abuse.

7.4.3. Violent and criminal behaviour

There is a considerable literature relating amphetamines to violence and crime (Grinspoon and Hedblom 1975). Some of the earliest reports came from Japan during the post-war methamphetamine epidemic. Masaki (1956) reported that more than half of 60 murderers convicted in Japan in May and June of 1954 were methamphetamine users. During the same period more than 10 000 people were arrested under the Awakening Drug Control Law, and more than half were found to be methamphetamine addicts. In the USA there was ambivalence about the connection between amphetamine use and criminal behaviour. As late as 1967, the President's Commission on Law Enforcement and Administration of Justice published a report that suggested that such a connection had not been proved, but events in Haight-Ashbury during the first methamphetamine epidemic soon changed that view. Carey and Mandel (1968, 1969) published insightful first-hand reports of the 'speed scene' in California in the 1960s. They reported more than 30 violent incidents involving users taking doses of 100–1000 mg of the drug daily (Carey and Mandel 1968). The actions were usually not premeditated and appeared motiveless and random to an outsider; for example, a man might strike his girlfriend or a parent hit a child for no obvious reason. The authors noted that violence was most likely to occur during the coming down ('crashing') phase of methamphetamine binges when the intensity of the user's irritability caused him to be intolerably angry and selfish.

Angrist and Gershon (1969) witnessed similar scenes in New York. They described the capricious nature of some of the attacks.

> The assaults were particularly frightening because of their unprovoked, grossly psychotic quality: One patient while walking down the street and feeling like the 'king of the universe' noticed a man walking near him. He had a fleeting idea that this stranger might be a homosexual but then his grandiosity reasserted itself; 'I decided he just didn't belong in my picture of things—so I took him out of the picture.' He then explained that he did this by carefully waiting until he was just abreast of the individual and then spinning and hitting him. This was repeated three or four times until he became frightened by what he was doing and came to Bellevue voluntarily. The second patient saw his roommate sleeping and felt that he 'looked dead'. He thereupon took a door handle and beat his head with it until restrained by a second roommate and taken to Bellevue. (Angrist and Gershon 1969)

Ellinwood (1971) gave detailed accounts of 13 murders committed by amphetamine users while intoxicated. In most instance paranoid thinking, emotional lability, panic, and lowered impulse control induced by the drug were instrumental factors. Logan *et al.* (1998) also described clear connections between methamphetamine-induced violence and fatalities.

Apart from the random violence induced by intoxication with amphetamines, the need for an ongoing supply of the drug can also lead to crime. The most common crime committed by amphetamine users is selling (dealing) the drug. As Tinklenberg and Stilman (1970) put it:

> The abuser's concerns increasingly narrow into the immediate present of procuring and using drugs as he becomes separate from the past and unconcerned about his

future. Any interference with these single-minded pursuits becomes an overwhelming threat, as his life has few other sources of satisfaction or meaning. Thus assaultative behaviour becomes more probable as the inhibitions to immediate action that usually come from recalling past experiences are minimized.

Grinspoon and Hedblom (1975) described three properties of amphetamine abuse that they regarded as mutually reinforcing risk factors for violent and criminal behaviour: First, high doses of amphetamines cause the subject to focus on immediate close-range stimuli. This may lead to impulsive reflex-like lashing out at innocent bystanders. The addict becomes apt to perceive anyone who seems to be interfering with his immediate drug-related pursuits as intolerably threatening. The result is a hugely increased risk of antisocial behaviour. A second factor is the ability of the drug to enhance the user's immediate awareness of stimuli, sensory cues, and visible objects or persons. This flood of sensory information is often accompanied by psychotic paranoia. Which information or person is to be trusted? He imagines that others are plotting against him and they must be attacked first. This risk is heightened by the typical lack of interpersonal relationships in the speed freak's life. This self-orientation can also be enormously damaging to the social fabric of the user's previous family or other friendships. When the speed freak's expectations, even if grossly unjustified, are perceived as rejected, he generally regards it as a personal affront, and vicious retaliation is common. A third risk factor is the psychomotor stimulant effects that are associated with amphetamine intoxication. Under the influence of the drug the user *must* do something, even if it is boring and repetitious 'punding'. If someone tries to interfere or disapprove of this behaviour, the addict may attack the perceived thwarter with murderous rage. Such violent retaliation helps to relieve the user's pent-up feelings of psychic and muscular tension. Accordingly, retribution accomplished by beatings, stabbings, shooting, and sometimes sadistic torture becomes a way of life. But because such amphetamine-related crime often occurs within the closed doors of the speed culture, such crime is largely ignored by the police and rarely leads to official arrests or convictions.

Morgan and Beck (1997) reported that 44 per cent of a group of 450 moderate to heavy crystal meth users in the USA reported violent behaviour as a result of using the drug, and methamphetamine-related violence occurs commonly in domestic disputes. Many methamphetamine users seen in psychiatric emergency rooms in the USA have reported long histories of aggression towards others (Szuster 1990).

Matters are no different in other countries. Connell (1958) was the first to systematically describe hostile or aggressive behaviour in amphetamine addicts in the UK. Corkery (2002) reported that in the year 2000 more than 6000 people in the UK were found guilty, cautioned, or fined for amphetamine-related offences. Klee and Morris (1994) examined the criminal activities of groups of heroin or amphetamine users in the UK. They found that heroin users' involvement in crime was related closely to their need to obtain money to purchase the drug, whereas the risk of amphetamine-related crime depended more closely on the frequency of drug use. Both groups reported similar overall rates of criminal activity.

7.4.4. Adverse effects of amphetamines on physical health

The physical condition of chronic amphetamine abusers is often very poor. Angrist and Sudilovsky (1978) surveyed the various ailments that amphetamine abusers may suffer. They are usually grossly malnourished and at the end of a 'run' are often markedly dehydrated. Chronic amphetamine users often exhibit repetitive chewing and teeth grinding, and as a result may experience dental problems and ulcers of the mouth and tongue caused by the constant irritation.

There are various adverse effects on the cardiovascular system, triggered by the excessive release of norepinephrine induced by the sympathomimetic actions of the drugs. After high doses these can include multiple extrasystoles, arrhythmias, hypertension, and heart block, and in overdose these can be lethal (Yu et al. 2003). In an early study, Waud (1938) described paroxysmal increases in heart rate and orthostatic hypotension (blood pressure dropping on rising). Waud's studies involved administering very large doses of Benzedrine. Subjects were asked to inhale the entire contents of two Benzedrine inhalers over a period of 4–6 hours. The total absorbed dose was estimated to be approximately 500 mg, vastly in excess of any normal medical or recreational use. It is not surprising that a rise in blood pressure lasting for up to 96 hours was observed, together with prolonged sleeplessness (for up to 3 days), a loss of appetite so severe as to cause weight loss, and a host of other adverse effects. Such a study design would not be ethically acceptable today! Chronic amphetamine use can also damage the heart muscle and the overlying myocardial membranes (Yu et al. 2003). Drug-induced damage to blood vessels in the brain can lead to stroke (Yu et al. 2003).

Skin ulcers and abscesses may be associated with compulsive scratching, but may also be related to poor hygiene in the intravenous injection of the drug in those users who self-inject. This can in turn lead to bacterial infections both at the site of injection and more generally, and such systemic infections can sometimes prove lethal. Poor injection techniques, including the shared use of needles, also increase the risk of viral infections, including HIV, hepatitis C, and hepatitis B. In addition, there is evidence that methamphetamine use has a suppressive effect on the immune system's ability to respond, making the user less able to counteract such infections (Yu et al. 2003).

As reviewed in Chapter 5, methamphetamine abuse is common among homosexual men who use the drug to increase sexual energy and stamina. Unfortunately, the propensity of the drug to lead to compulsive and sometimes reckless behaviour has also meant an associated increase in unprotected sex with multiple partners. This is causing considerable concern in the major cities of the USA where the incidence of HIV infection among the gay community is again on the rise (Frosch *et al.* 1996; Molitor *et al.* 1998). Apart from the risk of HIV or other viral infection as a result of risky sexual behaviour, there is also an increased risk of other sexually transmitted diseases, including syphilis and chlamydia, which are also currently increasing.

7.5. Overall conclusions

Millions of people have used moderate doses of amphetamine, usually taken in tablet form by mouth, for periods of many years without any overt signs of physical or mental harm. However, there is little doubt that those who become addicted to the chronic use of high doses of amphetamine or methamphetamine, especially those who self-inject, insufflate, or smoke the drugs, are likely to suffer a variety of serious adverse effects. Although there is little evidence for permanent drug-induced brain damage, amphetamines can cause long-lasting functional impairments in the function of monoamine neurons in the brain, particularly those using the neurotransmitter dopamine. This may also be accompanied by subtle long-term impairments in memory, attention, and decision-taking functions, which are essential for 'executive brain function', and these may recover only slowly after drug-taking ceases.

Chronic use can easily lead to dependence on the drug, and this in turn is often associated with a progressive break-up of social relationships, family life, and friendships. Laidler and Morgan (1997) have given a stark insight into the devastating effect that the methamphetamine epidemic in Hawaii has had on the social fabric of this close-knit community. Along with the 'self-orientation' of the amphetamine user come increased risks of impulsive irrational violence, criminal acts, and other forms of antisocial behaviour.

In addition, there are important physical health risks associated with long-term amphetamine use, and some of these can be life-threatening. The ability of the drugs to encourage risky sexual behaviour is particularly alarming in terms of the spread of HIV and other sexually transmitted diseases.

Overall the use of high-dose amphetamine is associated with an alarming series of adverse risks for both the user and those around him or her. One must hope that some way is found to halt the currently growing epidemic of methamphetamine abuse worldwide, lest, as in Hawaii (Apgar *Honolulu Star Bulletin*, 7 September 2003), it becomes the number one drug problem for many countries in the twenty-first century.

CHAPTER 8

Ecstasy

Ecstasy: 'an overwhelming feeling of joy or rapture'; 'an emotional or religious frenzy or trance-like state'

(*Concise Oxford Dictionary*, 9th edition 1995)

8.1. Chemistry and history

Ecstasy is the popular name for the amphetamine derivative 3,4-methylene-dioxy-methamphetamine (MDMA). Ecstasy and the related amphetamine derivative 3,4-methylemedioxy-amphetamine (MDA) (Fig. 2.1) are very widely used recreational drugs. A United Nations report estimated that there are as many as 8 million regular users worldwide, with an annual illicit manufacture of 125 tonnes (United Nations 2003).

Like the other amphetamines, ecstasy and MDA are relatively easy to manufacture. It is estimated that as much as 100 tonnes of the precursor chemical piperonyl methylketone (PMK) are smuggled into Europe every year—enough to make 100 million ecstasy tablets. A handful of Chinese chemical companies are almost the only major manufacturers of PMK, ostensibly for use in the perfumes industry, and the lucrative worldwide distribution network has fallen into the hands of Chinese Triad gangsters. Many small-scale ecstasy laboratories have sprung up around Europe, mainly in the Netherlands and Belgium and around Liverpool in the UK. A laboratory can cost as little as $8000 to set up and can be packed into a van to be moved from one location to another.

Because the US DEA exerts strict monitoring of the chemical precursors needed for ecstasy manufacture there are few illegal ecstasy laboratories in the USA. The DEA estimates that 80 per cent of US supplies of the drug are imported from the Netherlands, and in April 2004 US and Canadian police arrested a ring of dealers who had been importing bulk MDMA powder from the Netherlands into Canada for processing into tablets and subsequent trade across the US border (*Ottawa Citizen*, 5 April 2004). The expertise needed in MDMA production varies according to the route of synthesis (Nichols 2001). Clandestine production is easiest starting with PMK. Groups with access to PMK can make MDMA via a simple conversion process. Otherwise, MDMA can be synthesized from piperonal, isosafrole, or safrole. These primary precursor chemicals are produced in India, China, Poland, Germany, and increasingly elsewhere. Typically, safrole or isosafrole is first converted to PMK. The essential oil safrole occurs naturally as the primary constituent of oil of sassafras which is found in the root-bark of the US East Coast tree *Sassafras albidum* and in the above-ground woody parts of the South American tree *Ocotea pretiosa*. Safrole is also present in nutmeg (*Myristica fragrans*), dill, parsley seed, crocus, saffron, vanilla beans, and calamus.

As with any other mass market product, ecstasy is subject to the laws of supply and demand, and as the production of the drug has moved from a cottage industry to a sophisticated industrialized global business, the cost has come down dramatically—from more than £20 ($38) per tablet in the UK in 1990 to less than £3 ($5) in 2003. However, in the USA tighter controls on availability of precursors for ecstasy synthesis and stricter airport controls have restricted availability, and the average price of a tablet of ecstasy has risen in the past few years from about $10 a pill in 2001 to more than $15 a pill in 2004. But in Europe, with ecstasy costing not much more than a pint of beer or a packet of cigarettes, it is not surprising that consumption has soared. Tablets come in a variety of colours, shapes, and sizes, and have an average MDMA content of about 100 mg, although the content of active drug is highly variable and contamination with other drugs, notably MDA, methamphetamine, caffeine, and aspirin, is common.

MDA and MDMA are not new drugs. MDMA was first patented by the German pharmaceutical company Merck in 1914 as a chemical intermediate in the synthesis of other compounds. MDA was explored (unsuccessfully) as an appetite suppressant by Smith Kline and French under the name Amphedoxamine. Both MDA and MMDA were assessed during the 1950s by the US Army, who were interested in discovering a 'truth serum' to be used in interrogating enemy captives. During the late 1970s MMDA was widely used by psychotherapists attached to the Esalen Institute in California, who believed that it had 'substantial potential as an adjunct to psychoanalysis'. This pseudo-medical use spread quite widely among psychotherapists in the USA. By the early 1980s, over a thousand private psychotherapists in the USA were using MDMA in their clinical practice. MDMA was commonly known as 'Adam', an allusion to 'being returned to the natural state of innocence before guilt, shame and unworthiness arose'. It was used discreetly; no-one wanted a rerun of the excessive use of D-LSD and other psychedelic drugs by psychotherapists during the 1960s (Eisner 1989; Holland 2001a).

The psychedelic effects of these drugs have been known since the 1960s. MDA became one of the popular psychedelics in the American drug scene of the late 1960s. It was known as the 'hug drug', and MDA was said to stand for 'mellow drug of America'. Shulgin was among the first to report the psychedelic effects of ecstasy (MDMA) in the late 1960s, and it too became widely used among American university students (Shulgin 1986; Shulgin and Shulgin 2000). A survey of Stanford University undergraduates in 1987 revealed that 39 per cent had tried ecstasy, on average five times (Peroutka 1987).

MDMA was profiled by the *San Francisco Chronicle* (10 June 1984) as 'The Yuppie Psychedelic'. In *Newsweek*, J. Adler ('High on "ecstasy" ', 15 April 1985) likened his MDMA experience to 'a year of therapy in two hours'. *Harpers Bazaar* described MDMA as 'the hottest thing in the continuing search for happiness through chemistry'. Unsurprisingly, MDMA use soon spread beyond the couch and the clinic to the wider world. MDMA's now universal brand-name, 'ecstasy', was coined in 1981 by a member of a Los Angeles distribution network. The unnamed distributor apparently chose the name 'ecstasy' because 'it would sell better than calling it "Empathy". "Empathy" would be more appropriate, but how many people know what it means?' (Eisner 1989). Condemned by purists as a cynical marketing ploy, the brand-name 'ecstasy' is not wholly misleading (ecstasy: 'an overpowering emotion or exaltation; a state of sudden intense feeling, Rapturous delight. The frenzy of poetic inspiration. Mental transport or rapture from the contemplation of divine things' (*Oxford English Dictionary*)). Many first-time MDMA users do indeed become ecstatic. Some people report feeling truly well for the first time in their lives.

In July 1985, the US DEA, apparently alarmed by accounts of increasing addiction to ecstasy and by scientific reports that the related drug MDA might cause brain damage, placed an immediate ban on ecstasy and MDA. They were placed in the most restrictive category of all, reserved for damaging and addictive drugs without medical use. The effect of prohibition was to curtail research into the drug without changing the attitudes of recreational users. Indeed, the DEA's action helped to promote awareness of the drug in the mass media because a small group of people who were convinced of the value of ecstasy in psychotherapy sued the US DEA to try to prevent them from outlawing the drug. The controversy provided free advertising which made ecstasy use spread like wildfire throughout the USA. The temporary ban only lasted for a year; meanwhile a hearing was set up to decide what permanent measures should be taken against the drug. The case received much publicity and was accompanied by press reports advancing the kind of scare stories now current in Europe, which added to the pressure to make the ban permanent. One widely publicized report from the laboratory of the scientist George Ricaurte referred to evidence that the related drug, MDA, caused brain damage in rats and concluded that MDMA could cause brain damage in humans. The media indulged in horror scenarios of 'our kids' brains rotting by the time they were thirty', although there was no evidence that ecstasy caused brain damage in rats at the dosage levels used by humans. On the other side were the psychotherapists who gave evidence of the benefits of the drug, but they had failed to prepare their ground by carrying out scientifically acceptable trials and so their evidence was regarded as 'anecdotal' (Holland 2001a).

The case ended with the judge recommending that MDMA be placed in a less restrictive category, Schedule 3, which would have allowed it to be manufactured, to be used on prescription, and to be the subject of research. However, the recommendation was ignored by the DEA, which refused to back down and instead placed MDMA permanently in Schedule 1, where it has remained ever since. Despite this, some continued to urge the virtues of the drug in psychiatry. As Ann Shulgin put it: 'MDMA is penicillin for the soul; you don't give up penicillin when you see what it can do'.

MDA and ecstasy, together with other amphetamines, were made illegal in the UK in 1977 by adding them to the Misuse of Drugs Act 1971, even though ecstasy was not widely used in Europe until the late 1980s. It seems that the law-makers sought a blanket ban on all drugs with the basic amphetamine chemical structure. Ecstasy may have initially been brought to Europe by the followers of the eccentric Indian mystic Bhagwan Rajneesh, who used ecstasy as a source of 'self-enlightenment', when they dispersed from their base in Oregon after the Bhagwan and his followers were expelled in the late 1980s Some of the Bhagwan's followers may have brought ecstasy to the Spanish island of Ibiza during the winter of 1987–1988, where at the same time a new music movement was developing (Holland 2001a). People returning to the UK brought the musical concept along with the use of ecstasy, and so was born the rave scene in the UK. Raves were large gatherings of young people in warehouses or disused aircraft hangars where hundreds or thousands of people gathered and danced to the music until dawn or beyond. The scene was also called 'acid house' (reflecting the widespread use of another psychedelic drug, D-LSD) and developed its own symbols, such as the 'smiley face'. Warehouses were prepared secretly so as to avoid local people obtaining a court order to prevent the raves happening. Tickets were sold in advance without the address, but with a telephone number to ring on the night for instructions regarding a meeting place, such as a motorway service station, from where a convoy would proceed to the venue. Some entrepreneurs cashed in on the demand:

> As London's party culture absorbed ecstasy, the demand for underground warehouse parties grew, hundreds of people wanted to do the new wonder drug and dance all night. If you could not get any ecstasy then some old fashioned acid would do.
>
> Amongst the enthusiastic crowd who went to the parties was a young man called Tony Colston-Hayter. An imaginative, entrepreneurial technocrat with a relaxed attitude to legal formalities, he revolutionised the scene. He thought big. Instead of using dark, dodgy warehouses in London's docklands catering for a few hundred party-goers, why not organise parties for thousands of people in bigger venues?
>
> How he did it provides a fine illustration of free enterprise's ability to innovate by taking advantage of technological developments. The parties were attracting the attention of the police, who would raid them and close them down as soon as

they found out the location, unless the party was already in full swing, in which case they just turned people away rather than precipitate a riot.

Colston-Hayter reasoned that if he could get the people to the location in large numbers before the police arrived, the party would be unstoppable. He made use of a system called TVAR—Telephone Venue Address Releasing. The system worked as follows. During the day a production team would set up the venue, which could be a large warehouse or even an aircraft hangar. In total secrecy generators, sound systems, lighting, lasers, crash barriers, fire extinguishers, portaloos, merchandising stalls, food stands, soft drink stands and even a first aid room would be set up.

At a given time Colston-Hayter would use his cell phone to call a computer which would digitally record his spoken directions to a meeting point, usually somewhere on the M25 orbital motorway which circles London. The computerised system was linked to hundreds of phone lines.

The phone number would be printed on the tickets, and at a given hour would-be party-goers (and the police) would phone that number and within minutes thousands of callers from all over the South East of England would be in their cars and on the way to the meeting point. At the meeting point accomplices with cell phones would report back to him. Once a critical mass had been reached, and this might be as many as a thousand cars, he would record a new message giving the venue location. The sheer weight of numbers would render the police unable to stop the convoy of freedom loving party-goers heading for the party.

The profits on a party attended by over 10 000 people could be up to £50 000. The total turnover could easily be in the region of £250 000—fines for licensing offences were a maximum of £2000. (Saunders 1997)

Reynolds (1998), in his book *Energy Flash*, described what it was like to attend one of the largest of these events ever held, at Castlemorton Common in the West of England in May 1992.

> . . . arriving at the darkened common it quickly becomes apparent that the event has escalated beyond all expectations. Thanks to the Bank Holiday Monday's prolongation of the weekend, and exceptionally fine weather, Castlemorton is well on its way to becoming the biggest illegal rave in history. Estimates vary from twenty thousand to forty thousand present . . . . The midsummer night scene is somewhere between a medieval encampment and a Third World shanty town. The lanes are choked with caravans, buses, ex-military transports, gaudily painted horse drawn vehicles and hundreds of cars. The fields are jammed with a higgledy-piggledy throng of tents, pavilions, and eerie-looking fluorescent sculptures (the work of Sam Hegarty, resident artist for the Circus Irritant sound system).

> The Third World/medieval vibe is exacerbated by the bazaar atmosphere. Pedlars hawk their illicit wares, hollering 'get your acid!' or 'hash cookies for sale', propositioning with wraps of speed, magic mushroom pies and innumerable brands of ecstasy.

> After stumbling through the choc-a-bloc murk for what feels like an eternity, we finally make it to Spiral Tube's own enclosure, a Wild West style wagon circle of vans and trucks circumscribing a grassy dancefloor. While the event is free, in accordance with the Spiral credo 'no money, no ego', ravers are encouraged to give donations in order to keep 'the gennies' (electricity generators) running. Inside the circle, the scene is like a pagan gathering. With their amazing, undulating dance moves, it seems like the crowd has evolved into a single pulsating organism. Faces are contorted by expressions midway between orgasm and sobbing.

Opposition to raves was fierce, since people living up to 2 miles away could be kept awake all night. By 1990 the UK government had passed a new law which effectively put an end to these large gatherings. The law allowed for a fine of up to £20 000 and 6 months imprisonment for the organizers. Subsequently, further measures were enacted, including the Criminal Justice and Public Order Act 1994 which gave the police additional powers to stop people attending and to remove vehicles and sound equipment.

The result was to push ravers into dance clubs. The Hacienda in Manchester led the trend in 1988 with the now prevalent style—DJs who never spoke, but teased the dancers with their subtle 'scratching'—establishing the Manchester sound. From there 'clubbing on E' came to London, the rest of Europe, and eventually back to ecstasy's native California, as reported in the *San Francisco Examiner* in the winter of 1991: 'We were suddenly surrounded by these kids, moving here from England. They were coming here in droves and bringing with them a new sensibility, a new style of clothes.'

For a while in the early 1990s the rave dance fashion flourished in California, and as with so many other aspects of life the Southern Californians made it bigger and better than anywhere else. Entrepreneurs competed and outrivalled each other in organizing extravagant events, initially in illicit city or desert locations and eventually in legal sites, including one on a Disney facility and the largest rave party ever (17 000) on New Year's Eve 1992 at Knott's Berry Farm (Reynolds 1998). Reynolds describes one of these events:

> The most extravagant and over-the-top South California rave ever was probably Gilligan's Island, which took place in a Catalina casino-cum-ballroom. 1200 people were ferried over to the island in two ships. They took over the island, the cops wanted them to stop but they wouldn't. It was the pinnacle of Los Angeles rave—so outlawish, so brilliant . . . From then on, people were trying to match that vibe.

Unfortunately the ecstasy-driven Californian rave scene was soon overtaken by a far more dangerous drug, methamphetamine (speed) (see Chapter 5). The sudden growth of illicit methamphetamine laboratories in Southern California during the 1990s made it a cheap alternative to ecstasy. At rave dance events the methamphetamine-drugged participants no longer loved their fellow dancers but moved across the dance floor like zombies with vacant stares.

By this time ecstasy had reached nearly every corner of society in the UK, and by the winter of 1991–1992 demand had outstripped supply, partly because of some enormous police seizures. Dealers responded by selling any old tablet as ecstasy and no doubt made huge profits, but as a result many people had disappointing experiences and turned away from the drug. Analyses of tablets sold as ecstasy in Europe in the 1990s (Milroy *et al.* 1996; Saunders 1997) revealed that very few contained only ecstasy, and some contained none at all! Tablets were contaminated with a variety of drugs, including MDA, amphetamines, ephedrine, pseudo-ephedrine, and caffeine. About 10 per cent contained no active drug at all other than aspirin (Tylenol) or acetaminophen (paracetamol). Analysis of ecstasy tablets seized by police in the northwest of England during 2001 revealed an MDMA content ranging from 20 to 109 mg (Cole *et al.* 2002). A similar analysis of 33 capsules/tablets from US and UK suppliers in 1996 revealed that only half contained the normal dose of MDMA and many had no MDMA content at all (Saunders 1997). The high variability in MDMA dose is of course an important factor in determining its potential neurotoxic effects. Ecstasy is not manufactured by ethical pharmaceutical companies, and so there is no quality control. Up-to-date information on this topic is available at www.dancesafe.org/labtesting.

Many users turned to LSD instead, for the simple reason that the dose cannot be adulterated as it is microscopic (a thousand times smaller than a dose of MDMA) and is normally sold absorbed into a 'blotter', a tiny piece of paper too small to absorb active quantities of any other popular drug.

8.2. How do MDA and MMDA work in the brain?

Like other amphetamines, MDA and MMDA work indirectly by causing a release of monoamine neurotransmitters in the brain, but they target serotonin-containing nerves more potently than those containing dopamine or norepinephrine. These effects are illustrated by the data summarized in Table 8.1. Drugs were tested for their ability to cause release of each of the monoamines from nerve endings isolated from rat brain and studied in the test tube. The

Table 8.1 Monoamine-releasing properties of amphetamines in isolated rat brain nerve ending preparations

	Concentration for 50% maximum release (nM)		
	Dopamine release	Serotonin release	Norepinephrine release
D-Amphetamine	25	1765	7
D-Methamphetamine	25	736	12
DL-MDA	190	160	108
DL-MDMA	110	72	278

Data from Rothman and Baumann 2003.

monoamine stores were radiolabelled by incubating with a tracer amount of radiolabelled neurotransmitter which is selectively accumulated by the respective nerve ending transporter mechanisms (see Table 2.1). The preparations were then exposed to various concentrations of test drug in separate experiments to determine the concentration required to cause a release of each of the monoamines. Whereas amphetamine is 70 times more potent in displacing dopamine than serotonin, MDA and MMDA are as potent or more potent in displacing serotonin than dopamine. This reflects their relatively high affinity for the serotonin transporter mechanism, which is a feature of many other amphetamine-like drugs with benzene ring chemical substitutions, many of which also possess psychedelic properties.

MDMA-induced release of serotonin has also been demonstrated in intact animal brain by using the technique of implanted microdialysis probes, as described for amphetamine-induced dopamine release in Chapter 2, and by measurements of the depletion of serotonin stores in animal brain following drug administration (reviewed by Green *et al.* 2003). The involvement of the serotonin transporter was shown by the finding that pretreatment with the serotonin uptake inhibitor fluoxetine (Prozac®) greatly reduced the ability of MDMA to cause release of serotonin in rat brain (Mechan *et al.* 2002). MDMA also causes a release of dopamine in rat brain which can be measured by the microdialysis probe technique (Green *et al.* 2003), but whether this is due to a direct interaction with the dopamine transporter remains controversial. Some studies have indicated that the dopamine-releasing action of MDMA may be secondary to serotonin release. Dopamine release was not blocked by an inhibitor of dopamine uptake (Mechan *et al.* 2002) but it was attenuated by fluoxetine (Koch and Galloway 1997). MDMA also promotes norepinephrine release from brain slices or homogenate preparations *in vitro* (Table 8.1), but there is little evidence that this occurs in the intact brain *in vivo*. Even after chronic treatment with high doses of MDMA, there is little evidence of any depletion of norepinephrine stores in animal brain (Green *et al.* 2003).

That ecstasy-induced serotonin release in the brain plays a major role in the effects of the drug is supported by the observation that laboratory animals treated with ecstasy display the 'serotonin behavioural syndrome'. This was first described by Grahame-Smith (1971) following administration to rats of an inhibitor of monoamine oxidase together with the serotonin precursor L-tryptophan. It consists of hyperactivity, head weaving, forepaw treading, penile erection, salivation, and defecation. Ecstasy causes all of these acute behavioural features in rats in a dose-dependent manner (Green *et al.* 2003). The human equivalent of the 'serotonin syndrome' is also a real phenomenon; it can be produced by, for example, the inadvertent combination of serotoninergic drugs such as a monoamine oxidase inhibitor and a serotonin uptake inhibitor (e.g. fluoxetine) (Parrott 2002). The symptoms include hyperactivity, agitation, hyperpyrexia (fever), shivering, tremor, and slowing and increased heart rate. Several of these symptoms can be seen in a milder form in ecstasy users.

MDMA also interacts with a number of different monoamine receptors in the brain, but only at relatively high concentrations (1–100 μM). Such concentrations are unlikely to occur in human brain after the doses of MDMA normally used (1–2 mg/kg), although they may be achieved in animal studies after the administration of very high doses of the drug (10–20 mg/kg). Of potential relevance is the finding that MDMA can mimic serotonin at a receptor subtype known as 5-HT$_{2A}$. A variety of psychotomimetics drugs, including D-LSD and psilocybin, are thought to act via this receptor. However, MDMA rarely causes psychotomimetic reactions in human users.

The ability of MDMA to cause a rise in body temperature has proved to be an important factor in the acute toxicity of the drug, and is believed to have contributed to the deaths of some human users (see below). In rats and mice kept at normal room temperature (20–22°C) MDMA causes an increase in body temperature of 1–2°C (Green et al. 2003). This may not sound like a large increase, but in human terms it would be the equivalent of developing the sort of fever associated with a bad bout of influenza. The effect in laboratory animals depends on the ambient temperature. Rats kept in a cold room (10°C) show either no change or a small drop in body temperature in response to MDMA. However, animals kept in a warm environment (30°C) exhibit an exaggerated increase in body temperature (Gordon et al. 1991). The effect of MDMA on body temperature seems to be caused by its ability to enhance dopamine release in the brain rather than serotonin. The increase in body temperature elicited by MDMA in rats was not prevented by pretreatment with a serotonin receptor antagonist or the serotonin uptake inhibitor fluoxetine (Prozac®), but was blocked by pretreatment with dopamine receptor antagonists (Mechan et al. 2002). In this respect MDMA resembles methamphetamine, which also causes an increase in body temperature mediated via dopamine release (Bronstein and Hong 1995) (see Chapter 6).

8.3. What is the ecstasy experience like?

Pure MDMA salt is a white crystalline solid. It looks white and tastes bitter. The optimal adult dose of racemic MDMA is about 120–130 mg (about 2 mg/kg body weight). Pills sold in clubs often contain less. There are gender differences in response; proportionately to body weight, women are more sensitive than men to MDMA and so their optimal dosage may be lower. The preferentially metabolized (+)-enantiomer ('mirror image') of MDMA is more active, more stimulating, and more neurotoxic than the (−)-enantiomer. MDMA is usually taken orally as a tablet, capsule, or powder.

The effects of psychedelic drugs are intensely subjective and by definition are hard to describe in words. Although at the doses used in humans there is not a fully developed 'serotonin syndrome', some elements are present, including hyperactivity. Ecstasy also causes a highly unusual series of changes in consciousness. It has been described as an 'empathogen' because it can promote an extraordinary clarity of introspective self-insight, together with a deep love of self and a no less emotionally intense empathetic love of others. MDMA also acts as a euphoriant. The euphoria is usually gentle and subtle; but is sometimes profound.

The experience is usually intensely pleasurable, with heightened awareness of sensory stimuli, a breakdown of normal social barriers and inhibitions, and increased empathy. In addition, there is an amphetamine-like stimulant effect which allows the user to stay awake and indulge in energetic activities for long periods of time. The onset of action can take 20–60 minutes, with peak effects usually occurring 60–90 minutes after ingestion, and the primary effects last for 3–5 hours. Alexander Shulgin was one of the first to describe the subjective effects of the drug, and he introduced many others to it. Shulgin experienced somewhat mixed results in testing the drug on himself, but described some of his experiences as follows. After taking a dose of 100 mg:

> My mood was light, happy, but with an underlying conviction that something significant was about to happen. There was a change in perspective both in the near visual field and in the distance. My usually poor vision was sharpened. I saw details in the distance that I could not normally see. After the peak experience had passed, my major state was one of deep relaxation. I felt that I could talk about deep or personal subjects with special clarity, and I experienced some of the feeling one has after the second martini, that one is discoursing brilliantly and with particularly acute analytical powers.

After taking 120 mg:

> I felt absolutely clean inside, and there is nothing but pure euphoria. I have never felt so great or believed this to be possible. The cleanliness, clarity and marvelous feeling of solid inner strength continued throughout the rest of the day, and evening, and through the next day. I am overcome by the profundity of the experience, and how much more powerful it was than previous experiences, for no apparent reason, other than a continually improving state of being. All the next day I felt like a 'citizen of the universe' rather than a citizen of the planet, completely disconnecting time and flowing easily from one activity to the next. (Shulgin and Shulgin 2000)

Some young ecstasy users also found their first experience of the drug profoundly memorable (extracted from www.interdope.com):

> I'd have to say that in all of my eighteen years it was the most beautiful moment of my life.

> It was the most euphoric experience of my life.

The peak was the most mind blowing experience I have ever had.

It was as if I was in heaven. It was the best experience I have ever had!

It was one of the greatest experiences of my life.

I lived in a pure state of euphoria that night. It was the best feeling I had ever had in my life.

One of the unusual features of the MDMA experience is that the drug encourages social contacts and breaks down emotional barriers. This is the aspect most praised by those psychotherapists who have used the drug as an adjunct to normal therapy.

The MDMA experience in the context of a rave dance event has been well described by Simon Reynolds, whose book *The Energy Flash* (Reynolds 1998) gives an excellent account of the remarkable growth of the rave dance culture in the UK in the 1990s and the impact it had on youth culture.

> At a rave, the emotional outpouring and huggy demonstrativeness is a huge part of the MDMA experience (which is why ravers use the term 'loved up'), but the intimacy is dispersed into a general bonhomie: you bond with the gang you came with, but also people you've never met. . . .
>
> The blitz of noise and lights at a rave tilts the MDMA experience towards the drug's purely sensuous and sensational effects. With its mild trippy, pre-hallucinogenic feel, ecstasy makes colours, sounds, smells, tastes and tactile sensations more vivid . . . . The experience combines clarity and a limpid soft-focus radiance. . . .
>
> All music sounds better on E—crisper and more distinct, but also engulfing in its immediacy. House and techno sound especially fabulous. The music's emphasis on texture and timbre enhances the drug's mildly synaesthetic effects; so that sounds seem to caress the listener's skin . . . . Organised around the absence of crescendo or narrative progression, rave music instills a pleasurable tension, a rapt suspension that fits perfectly with the pre-orgasmic plateau of the MDMA high.

The effects of ecstasy on sexual function are subtle. MDMA is sensuous in its effects without being distinctively pro-sexual; it is more of a hug-drug than a love-drug. However, MDMA's capacity to dissolve a lifetime's social inhibitions, prudery, and sexual hang-ups means that lovemaking while under its spell is not uncommon. In men, orgasm is more intense than normal but is delayed; MDMA retains a residual sympathomimetic activity, triggering a detumescence of the male organ. To ease MDMA-induced performance difficulties, flagging Romeos increasingly combine ecstasy with Viagra.

It is easy to understand why ecstasy has proved so popular with young people. However, not every ecstasy experience is positive; some 25 per cent of users report having had at least one adverse reaction, when unpleasant feelings and bodily sensations predominated (Davison and Parrott 1997). Minor adverse reactions are also common, but are generally short-lived. These include mydriasis (dilated pupils), photophobia (discomfort in bright lighting), headache, sweating, tachycardia (rapid heart beat), bruxism (grinding of teeth), trismus (uncomfortable tightening of jaw muscles), and loss of appetite.

8.4. How dangerous is ecstasy?

8.4.1. Ecstasy-related deaths

Until the late 1980s the use of ecstasy was not controlled by legislation, but since then it has been portrayed as a dangerous narcotic on both sides of the Atlantic and placed in the highest category of harmful drugs, along with heroin and cocaine. This was a reaction partly to the widespread use of ecstasy on college campuses in the USA during the 1980s and partly to the first reports of ecstasy-related deaths among young people. The banning of legal ecstasy was later reinforced by scientific evidence which appeared to show that the drug could cause irreversible brain damage in both animals and humans.

The first reports of ecstasy-related deaths appeared in the USA in 1987 (Dowling et al. 1987) and in Europe a few years later (Milroy 1999). In the early cases drug-induced hyperthermia (abnormally elevated body temperature) appeared to be the principal cause. All those who died had been admitted to hospital with high temperatures (40–43 °C), which lead to damage to the liver, heart, and other organs. In an attempt at harm reduction, advice was given that dancers at rave events should take time out, go to a 'chill-out' area, and drink plenty of liquid. Unfortunately, some took this advice too literally; by 1993 deaths of ecstasy users from water intoxication began to be reported (Milroy 1999). Kalant (2001) surveyed reports on 87 ecstasy-related deaths in the world literature at that time and found that hyperthermia was the most common single cause (30 out of the total). An analysis of the true risks of fatal intoxication with ecstasy is difficult to make. The unnecessary death of each young person is of course a personal tragedy for their family and loved ones, and the media have given these events prominent cover and used them to convey the message that ecstasy is a deadly poison. However, the data need to be looked at in perspective. It has been estimated that more than 5000 elderly people die each year in the USA from gastric bleeding caused by over-use of aspirin-like medicines (Tamblyn et al. 1996). The rare deaths attributed to ecstasy need to be considered in relation to the very large number of users of the drug. During the 4-year period 1997–2000 a total of 81 deaths in England and Wales were reported to be related to ecstasy use (Schifano et al. 2003). However, post-mortem analysis revealed that most of those who died had been taking other drugs (prescribed and non-prescribed) at the same time as ecstasy; more than half (59 per cent) had taken heroin or a related opiate. Indeed, most of the dead were known to the welfare or medical services as drug addicts, and typically they died at home rather than at a rave dance event. Only six of the total of 81 appeared to have died after taking only ecstasy. A case series in New York City studied 19 366 deaths between January 1997 and July 2000 for which post-mortem toxicological analysis was available (Gill *et al.* 2002). Only 22 of these were considered to be ecstasy related. As in the UK, the presence of other drugs was common in the ecstasy-related cases: heroin or other opiates in 32 per cent, alcohol in 32 per cent, ketamine in 27 per cent, and cocaine in 22 per cent.

A potentially serious adverse effect of ecstasy was pointed out by Setola *et al.* (2003) who reported that the drug had an appreciable affinity for 5-HT_{2B} receptors and could promote a proliferation of cells in human heart valve tissue culture. Other drugs that have this property, notably the anti-obesity drug fenfluramine, have been found to be associated with potentially lethal heart valve disease (see Chapter 3). To date, however, there is no epidemiological evidence for an increased risk of heart valve disease in current or previous ecstasy users.

8.4.2. Tolerance and dependence

In one of the first descriptions of human reactions to ecstasy, Shulgin (1986) commented: 'MDMA does not lend itself to overuse because its most desirable effects diminish with frequency of use'.

This proved to be an astute observation. Parrott (2005) reviewed his own surveys of ecstasy users and various reports published by others. It was apparent that there were clear differences in the pattern of drug consumption between novice users and those who were more experienced. Whereas novices used one or two tablets per session, more experienced users took two or three tablets and heavy users (lifetime use more than 100 tablets) took more than three tablets in each session. Although this provides evidence for tolerance, there was little to suggest that many ecstasy users become dependent on the drug, although for some users the association of the drug with the rave dance/club scene may become a way of life.

A more sinister aspect of tolerance to ecstasy is that the use of increasing doses may tend to exaggerate the psychostimulant effects of the drug, believed to be due largely to dopamine release in the brain. As one close observer of the ecstasy scene described it:

> By 1992, many hardcore 'veterans', who'd gotten into raving only a few years earlier and were often still in their teens, had increased their intake to three, four, five, or more pills per session. They were locked into a cycle of going raving once or twice a week, weekend after weekend. It was at this point that ecstasy's serotonin-depletion effect came into play. Even if you take pure MDMA each and every time, the drug's blissful effects fade fast, leaving only a jittery, amphetamine-like rush. In hardcore, this speedfreak effect was made worse as ravers necked more pills in a futile and misguided attempt to recover the long-lost bliss of yore. The physical

side-effects—hypertension, racing heart—got worse, and so did the darkside paranoia. (Reynolds 1998, p. 192)

The author showed a remarkable insight into the possible neurochemistry underlying tolerance to ecstasy. Animal studies indeed show that the drug can cause a profound temporary impairment of serotonin function in the brain, while such changes do not occur to the same extent with dopamine-related functions (Green *et al.* 2003). The possibility that the amphetamine-like effects of ecstasy become more prominent in heavy users of the drug may explain why some heavy ecstasy users indulge in 'bingeing' (Parrott 2005) (see Chapter 5). During a binge users may take several tablets at once, or take repeated tablets during a session, or both. The binge may last for up to 48 hours, usually without sleep or food, and can involve taking up to 20 ecstasy tablets. Some binge users 'snort' the powdered drug or inject it. These heavy users of ecstasy certainly show signs of becoming dependent on the drug, and many suffer harmful effects— days off with illness, loss of appetite, weight loss, and depressive experiences. Sumnall and Cole (2005) undertook a meta-analysis of 25 published surveys indicating self-reported depression in ecstasy users and concluded that it was a common phenomenon, although the effects were relatively small.

Animal studies have added little to our understanding of tolerance to and dependence on ecstasy. Whether experimental animals will readily self-administer a psychoactive drug is one widely used test of whether it is likely to prove addictive in humans. By this criterion ecstasy is not likely to be addictive, since animals do not usually self-administer it. However, under special experimental conditions animals can be taught to self-administer ecstasy. Fantegrossi *et al.* (2004) trained monkeys to self-administer ecstasy by first teaching them to self-administer cocaine (which they do very readily), and then switching to ecstasy. The animals continued to self-administer small doses of ecstasy for up to 18 months, although their consumption gradually went down during this period, which did not happen in animals trained to self-administer cocaine.

8.4.3. Neurotoxicity in animals

There is large scientific literature on the effects of ecstasy on animal brain, focusing largely on the long-term damaging effects that the drug can have on serotonin-containing nerves (Ricaurte *et al.* 2000; Green *et al.* 2003). The literature is complex and often confusing, partly because there are marked differences in the effects of ecstasy in different species (the drug has little effect on the serotonin system in mouse brain, but rats, guinea pigs, and monkeys are sensitive), but also because most animal studies used doses of ecstasy that were far higher than those taken by human drug users. Again, this resembles the many studies on amphetamine/methamphetamine neurotoxicity in animals which used excessively high sublethal doses (see Chapter 7). In addition, in most animal studies ecstasy was administered by injection rather than orally, and this leads to faster drug absorption and higher peak levels in blood than the slower oral route employed by most human users. The use of high doses of ecstasy in animal studies is usually justified by the 'interspecies scaling' model of drug metabolism (Ricaurte et al. 2000). Briefly stated, this takes account of the fact that smaller animals such as the rat generally inactivate drugs more rapidly than humans. Thus, for example, in rats one generally needs to administer a dose that is 5–10 times higher than the normal human dose in order to generate drug levels in the rat blood comparable to those seen in humans. However, there is little comparative information available on the way in which ecstasy is metabolized in animals and humans, and this approach has been criticized. Furthermore, a comparison of the behavioural and other actions of amphetamines in animals and humans suggested that, for this group of compounds, there was a much smaller gap between effective animal and human doses than that predicted by the normal scaling rules (Grilly and Loveland 2001). Although this review did not include ecstasy, it is likely to follow similar rules as it is chemically similar to the other amphetamines.

Nevertheless, it is clear that high doses of ecstasy do cause damage to serotonin nerves in both rat and monkey brain. The drug causes a depletion of brain levels of serotonin itself, as might be expected from its mode of action as a serotonin releaser. But in addition there is a long-lasting reduction in other neurochemical markers of serotonin nerves, including the biosynthetic enzyme tryptophan hydroxylase and the serotonin transporter mechanism, suggesting damage to the serotonin-containing nerve terminals. Both of these remain depleted for weeks or months after a single dose or course of doses of ecstasy, although there is a slow recovery to near-normal values that may take up to a year to complete (Green et al. 2003).

Further direct evidence for drug-induced damage to serotonin nerves came from anatomical studies of animal brain using selective staining methods to visualize serotonin nerve fibres; these also showed a marked depletion of serotonin-containing nerves in all brain regions. However, the nerve cell bodies from which the serotonin fibres emanate do not appear to be irreversibly damaged; what the drug seems to do is to 'prune' the fibres in their terminal regions. This means that slow recovery is possible as the remaining nerve cells and fibres regenerate. However, while some brain regions may recover a normal or even supernormal regrowth of serotonin fibres, other brain regions, such as the cerebral cortex, that are further away from the serotonin nerve cells in the brainstem may take much longer or may never recover to normal (Green et al. 2003). In monkeys treated with neurotoxic doses of ecstasy, the density of serotonin-containing fibres was only 50–60 per cent of control values 7 years later (Hatzidimitriou et al. 1999). Scheffel et al. (1998) used a brain imaging technique and the radioactively labelled drug $[^{11}C](+)McN5652$ to label the serotonin transporter. Using this technique they could monitor the ecstasy-induced depletion of serotonin transporter sites and their recovery in the brains of baboons treated with neurotoxic doses of ecstasy. Significant reductions were observed in all brain regions during the first 40 days after drug treatment, but by 13 months serotonin transporter densities had recovered to levels above baseline in brainstem and hypothalamus, although they remained significantly depleted in the cerebral cortex.

The effects of ecstasy on brain serotonin systems are dose dependent. Most studies have used a regime of twice-daily injections of the drug for up to 4 days, and the doses needed to cause long-lasting damage to serotonin nerves are approximately 20 mg/kg in rats and 4 mg/kg in monkeys—a far more extreme exposure to the drug than the 1–2 mg/kg oral doses taken by most human ecstasy users. Although these dose regimes have been justified on the basis of 'interspecies scaling' (Ricaurte *et al.* 2000), the validity of this model for ecstasy studies is questionable. Injection of a dose of 10 mg/kg of ecstasy in rhesus monkeys led to plasma drug levels 10 times higher than those seen in human subjects. It is also possible that the neurotoxicity of ecstasy in animal studies is caused by the formation of toxic metabolites; the drug does not cause damage to serotonin nerves when injected directly into rat brain (Estaban *et al.* 2001). Since rats and humans metabolize the drug in different ways, this is another reason to suggest that the animal studies may not reliably predict the human toxicity of the drug (de la Torre and Farré 2004).

Perhaps a more realistic model is to allow the animal to self-administer the drug. Fantegrossi *et al.* (2004) reported a study in rhesus monkeys in which the animals were trained to self-administer ecstasy intravenously by pressing a lever. The animals were allowed two periods of 1 hour each day for drug administration. On average they injected a dose of 2–4 mg/kg in each session, not much different from the normal human dose. The experiment continued for 18 months, although the animals showed a decreasing rate of self-administration during this time. Two months after the end of the self-administration period the animals were subjected to various brain imaging studies and their brains were examined post-mortem for signs of damage to the serotonin nerves. None of these animals showed any signs of serotonin neurotoxicity.

The mechanisms involved in the neurotoxic actions of ecstasy remain unclear, but they seem to be closely related to the ability of the drug to cause hyperthermia (Green *et al.* 2003). In rats this is in turn dependent on the ambient temperature during drug administration; at temperatures below 24°C there was no significant long-term depletion of brain serotonin, whereas significant depletion was observed at ambient temperatures of 26°C or above (Malberg and Seiden 1998). Drugs that lower body temperature can protect animals against long-term ecstasy-induced damage to serotonin nerves (Green *et al.* 2003).

The effects of ecstasy appear to be selective for serotonin nerves. Although the drug is a substrate for uptake into dopamine-containing nerves and causes a release of dopamine that contributes in part to the overall drug action, there is little evidence for any lasting damage to brain dopamine systems. In a classic mistake, the laboratory of George Ricaurte, who has cultivated a prominent media image for his strong views on the neurotoxicity of ecstasy, claimed to have observed severe damage to dopamine neurons in monkey brain after injecting ecstasy (three injections of 2 mg/kg in each session) (Ricaurte *et al.* 2002). The authors warned of the dangers of drug-induced Parkinson's disease in ecstasy users, and the report gained much publicity. However, it turned out that the animals had received methamphetamine in error and not ecstasy, and the group was subsequently forced to retract (Ricaurte *et al.* 2003).

8.4.4. Is ecstasy a serotonin neurotoxin in human users?

The question of whether the animal data on the neurotoxic actions of ecstasy are relevant to human users of the drug is vexed. The issue is clouded by politics as well as science. Governments on both sides of the Atlantic, but especially in the USA, have sought to use scientific evidence to defend their classification of ecstasy as a dangerous narcotic. In the USA the National Institute on Drug Abuse (NIDA) has provided generous research grants to scientists working on the possible toxic effects of ecstasy. For example, the neurologist George Ricaurte and his wife Una McCann and their colleagues at Johns Hopkins University, have received tens of millions of US dollars in research grants from NIDA over more than a decade. They have been particularly willing to take a strong stand in portraying ecstasy as a 'potent serotonin neurotoxin' (McCann *et al.* 2000) and have cultivated media attention to their research. NIDA in turn has used Ricaurte and McCann's research results in their own campaign of information about ecstasy, portraying it as a dangerous narcotic capable of causing irreversible brain damage.

What are the facts? Clearly, it is not possible to make direct measurements of serotonin or markers of the integrity of serotonin nerves in human brain. Therefore various indirect approaches must be adopted. One of these involves measurements of the serotonin breakdown product 5-hydroxylindoleacetic acid (5-HIAA) in the cerebrospinal fluid (CSF) which bathes nerve cells in the brain and spinal cord. The level of 5-HIAA can be used to indicate whether serotonin mechanisms are functioning normally. Unfortunately, CSF samples are taken by lumbar puncture from the spinal cord rather than the brain, and levels of 5-HIAA are known to be influenced by diet, age, gender and other factors. Whereas the data from Ricaurte's group indicated that CSF 5-HIAA levels were abnormally low in ecstasy users (McCann *et al.* 1994), another group failed to find any such alterations (Peroutka *et al.* 1987). Another approach has been to use brain imaging with radiolabelled McN5652 as a way of assessing the integrity of the serotonin transporter in the brains of ecstasy users. One such study from Ricaurte's laboratory attracted much attention (McCann et al. 1998b).It compared 14 regular users of ecstasy who had abstained for at least 3 weeks with 15 normal controls. The results appeared to show that there were major losses of serotonin transporter sites in the brains of the ecstasy users. The startling images of brains that appeared to have holes in them were seized upon by NIDA, who used thesm in their own campaigns, showing the images under the title 'Your Brain on Ecstasy' (of course the images did not show 'holes in the brain' but, rather, an apparent loss of this marker for serotonin nerves). The McCann et al. (1998b) study was referred to in the official report of the US Sentencing Commission in 2001 which led to longer prison sentences for ecstasy-related offences. The Director of NIDA, Alan Leshner, stated to a Senate hearing in July 2001: 'There is across-the-board agreement that brain damage does occur . . . Research has unequivocally shown that MDMA literally damages nerve cells'.

However, the McCann et al. (1998b) study has been criticized on several grounds (Kish 2002). The tracer $[^{11}C](+)$McN5652 is not easy to use; it has a high level of non-specific binding to sites other than the serotonin transporter, making it difficult to measure the small amount of 'specific' binding. The individual results in the McCann study were highly variable, scattered over more than a 30-fold range between the lowest and highest values in the controls. The authors transformed the data into log units to reduce this variability, but the validity of such a transformation is questionable. Nevertheless, further studies using the same tracer have yielded more consistent results and have confirmed that there is a reduction in serotonin transporter density in several brain regions in current ecstasy users (Buchert et al. 2004), although the reduction appears to be less severe than the 50–75 per cent loss originally implied by McCann et al. (1998b). Women appear more susceptible than men; indeed in a study by Reneman et al. (2001), who used a different tracer ($[^{123}I]2\beta$-carbomethoxy-3β(4-iodophenyl) tropane ($[^{123}I]\beta$-CIT)), statistically significant reductions in transporter densities were only seen in the female subject group, and not in men. Small reductions in $[^{123}I]\beta$-CIT binding in current ecstasy users were also reported by Semple et al. (1999). However, $[^{123}I]\beta$-CIT is not considered to be a reliable marker for serotonin transporter sites since it is also recognized with high affinity by the dopamine transporter in brain, and in animals it does not appear to be capable of labelling the low density of serotonin transporter sites in the cerebral cortex (Heinz and Jones 2000). Both of the more recent imaging studies (Reneman et al. 2001; Buchert et al. 2004) also included groups of subjects who had stopped using ecstasy; no reductions in serotonin transporter densities were found in these, suggesting that the changes observed in current users are reversible. In summary, the neuroimaging data provide evidence for modest reversible changes in serotonin neurons in response to ecstasy, although it is not clear that these are accompanied by actual damage to serotonin-containing nerve fibres. This conclusion is closely similar to that reached for human imaging studies of methamphetamine-induced changes in dopamine function and dopamine transporter levels (see Chapter 7).

An alternative approach to assessing the functional state of serotonin mechanisms in the brain is to evoke a hormonal response with serotonin-related drugs. Serotonin is involved in the hypothalamic–pituitary–adrenal axis which regulates hormonal responses to stress. The exact role of serotonin is not clear, but it is involved in the secretion of the hormones prolactin, cortisol, and growth hormone. Pharmacological challenges have been used to assess serotonin hormonal function in ecstasy users. Gerra *et al.* (1998) found that prolactin and cortisol responses to the serotonin-releasing agent fenfluramine were significantly reduced in ecstasy users, and McCann *et al.* (1997b) made similar observations using the drug metachlorophenylpiperazine as a serotonin releaser. Thus these studies support the conclusion that serotonin mechanisms are blunted in the brains of ecstasy users.

Less direct evidence has sought to relate impairments in memory tests and sleep disturbances in ecstasy users to impaired serotonin function (McCann *et al.* 2000). However, the question of whether cognitive impairments are consistently found in ecstasy users and whether they persist after drug use is stopped is controversial, and some have challenged the validity of these and other neuropsychological assessments (McGuire 2000; Parrott 2002). Claims that ecstasy use might precipitate long-term psychiatric illness also seem to be based on small numbers of case studies. McGuire (2000) concluded:

> Clinical case reports suggest that regular MDMA use can be associated with chronic psychiatric symptoms which persist after the cessation of drug use. However, it is difficult to determine whether MDMA use is directly responsible, triggers symptoms in subjects predisposed to mental illness, or is incidental. In any event, severe long term psychiatric disturbances following MDMA use seem uncommon relative to the large numbers of people who use MDMA. Neuropsychological comparisons of regular MDMA users and controls suggest that MDMA may be associated with memory deficits, with other cognitive processes unaffected, although there have been only a limited number of studies, each using different methods of assessment. It is assumed that these putative and clinical sequelae are secondary to an effect of MDMA on brain serotoninergic function, but the relationship between psychological and biological changes in MDMA users has yet to be determined.

However, others disagree. Morgan (2000) reviewed the literature on the persistent psychological effects of ecstasy and concluded that chronic heavy recreational use of the drug is associated with sleep disorders, depressed mood, elevated anxiety, impulsiveness and hostility, and selective impairment of episodic and working memory and attention. The cognitive deficits may persist for 6 months or more of abstinence, but all symptoms appear to remit within 6–12 months.

It seems reasonable to conclude that ecstasy causes a temporary depletion of brain serotonin stores and some degree of downregulation of serotonin function, although there is little evidence that these changes are irreversible. The conclusion that some disruption of normal serotonin function occurs after drug use is consistent with the common observation that for several days after taking ecstasy users complain of depressed mood and lethargy ('sometimes referred to as the 'midweek blues') (Parrott 2002). Serotonin is known to be importantly involved in the control of mood; modern antidepressant drugs such as fluoxetine (Prozac®) act by blocking the serotonin transporter and thus enhancing the levels of serotonin available at the synapse. Midweek low moods with problems of concentration or memory difficulties are common in ecstasy users, but these are transient changes with mood reverting to normal within 7 days (Parrott and Lasky 1998). Regular users of ecstasy can become tolerant to the drug, requiring increasing doses to achieve the desired effect (Parrott 2005). Reynolds (1998), an acute observer and participant in the ecstasy dance culture, describes the phenomenon with his own perceptive neurochemical interpretations as follows:

> It takes about a week for serotonin levels to normalize. Taking ecstasy is like going on an emotional spree, spending your happiness in advance. With irregular use, such extravagance isn't a problem. But with sustained and excessive use, the brain's serotonin levels become seriously depleted, so that it takes around six weeks' abstinence from MDMA to restore normal levels.
>
> If you take E every day, within a few days the blissful, empathetic, serotonin glow wears off, leaving only the speedy, dopamine buzz; this in-built diminishing returns syndrome is one reason why MDMA isn't considered physically addictive. The honeymoon period with ecstasy that most ravers enjoy can, however, create an emotional addiction, in so far as normal life seems dreary compared to the loved-up abandon of the weekend. This is when ecstasy's potential for abuse enters the picture. Because the original blissed-out intensity of the early experiences never really returns, users are tempted to increase the dose, which only increases the speediness and amplifies the unpleasant side effects. Serious hedonists get locked into a punishing cycle of weekend excess followed by the inevitable brutal midweek crash.

The question of how damaging ecstasy may be to brain serotonin neurons remains open. At an international conference held in 2000 experts from various disciplines were asked to give their answer to the question: Is MDMA a human neurotoxin? Fifteen of the participants submitted brief answers to this question, and they were split almost exactly equally between those who were convinced that there was some evidence of long-lasting adverse effects, and those who believed the evidence to be unconvincing. Several mentioned the absence of glial cell reactions in animal brains after high-dose ecstasy as evidence against organic brain damage (neural damage in the brain usually triggers a proliferation of non-neural glial cells.) (Turner and Parrott 2000).

8.4.5. Does ecstasy have potential medical uses?

During the 1970s and early 1980s ecstasy was widely used by psychotherapists in the USA, and many believed strongly in its positive therapeutic benefits as an adjunct to psychotherapy. Some US psychiatrists and psychoanalysts described ecstasy as the 'penicillin' of their field—a new wonder-drug. Indeed, when the US DEA announced its intention to schedule ecstasy in July 1984, it faced a formal legal challenge from a well-organized group of respected physicians (Grob 2000; Holland 2001a). However, the DEA did not wait for the outcome of this challenge, and in July 1985 temporarily placed ecstasy in the highest category, Schedule I, which is reserved for the most dangerous drugs of abuse that have no recognized medical uses. Nevertheless, three public hearings took place, presided over by the DEA Administrative Law Judge Francis Young. Many therapists, psychiatrists, and patients came forward to plead for a less restrictive scheduling which would allow the continued use of ecstasy on a prescription basis for medical research. The resulting testimony filled 10 volumes. Most people were stunned by Judge Young's recommendation on 22 May 1986.

> The record now assembled contains much more material about MDMA than the Agency was aware of when it initiated this proceeding . . . The evidence of record does not establish that MDMA has a high potential for abuse. It cannot be placed in Schedule I because it does have a currently accepted medical use in treatment and it does have accepted safety for use under medical supervision. Based on this record it is the recommended decision of the administrative law judge that MDMA should be placed in Schedule III.

However, the victory was short-lived, as the DEA overrode the recommendation of their own judge and placed ecstasy permanently in Schedule I. This decision was again challenged by advocates of the medical uses of ecstasy, and they won in a federal district court. The DEA again overruled this judgment, corrected legal procedural problems identified by the court, and confirmed the Schedule I status of the drug, where it has remained to this day.

The problem for advocates of a revival of medical use of ecstasy is that there is little rigorous scientific evidence for its alleged therapeutic benefits. During the period of its use by psychotherapists the concept of controlled clinical trials in psychiatry or psychotherapy was not a familiar one. Thus the usefulness of ecstasy rested largely on word of mouth and anecdote. As Alan Leshner, former director of NIDA, liked to say: 'The plural of anecdote is not data'.

Some advocates of the therapeutic benefits of ecstasy never gave up. Rick Doblin started taking psychedelic drugs as a student and became convinced of the healing power of LSD and ecstasy. He helped to coordinate the legal challenge to the DEA in 1985, and later helped to form the Multidisciplinary Association for Psychedelic Studies (MAPS) based in Sarasota, Florida, which has lobbied for the revival of ecstasy and other psychedelic drugs as therapeutic agents. Professor Julie Holland of New York University has also been a long-standing supporter of the therapeutic uses of ecstasy, and is an authority on the topic. She edited the book *Ecstasy: The Complete Guide* (Holland 2001b) which marshals the evidence in favour of a revival of interest in ecstasy as a prescription medicine.

MAPS eventually managed to persuade the US Food and Drug Administration to approve a clinical trial of ecstasy in patients with post-traumatic stress disorder (PTSD). However, the spurious paper published by Ricaurte *et al.* (2002) claiming that ecstasy might cause Parkinson's disease-like damage to monkey brain sparked a furore that prevented this trial from starting. Ricaurte's findings also damaged the chances of a similar clinical trial which was due to start in Spain in patients with PTSD. Ricaurte himself lectured in Spain about the dangers of ecstasy. However, the finding that the data in the paper published by Ricaurte *et al.* (2002) were not due to ecstasy but to methamphetamine, given in error, and the subsequent retraction (Ricaurte *et al.* 2003) changed the climate of opinion. In 2003 approval was again given for a trial of ecstasy in PTSD in North Carolina, and finally in February 2004 the DEA granted a special license to dispense ecstasy for this trial (Check 2004).

PTSD seems an obvious condition for further research with ecstasy. As Julie Holland put it:

> PTSD is a particular anxiety-related illness in people who have undergone an extreme traumatic event that negatively affects their lives. Rape victims, people who have been assaulted, victims of torture and war may all be helped by MDMA-assisted psychotherapy. MDMA allows people to revisit the trauma with much less anxiety than usual and to work through what has occurred in a non-threatening context, perhaps allowing for a measure of forgiveness and acceptance to occur for the event. Uncovering the repressed memories and speaking about them calmly and openly is a first step toward clinical improvement in PTSD . . . If MDMA has any chance of being transformed into an FDA-approved medication, it is likely to be with this clinical indication. (D. Adams and B. Fulton, *Salt Lake City Weekly*, 30 September 2004)

PTSD is not the only condition that may be helped by ecstasy. Holland (2001b) contains reviews of other possible applications in the treatment of depression and schizophrenia, and in psychotherapy more generally. However, given the way in which ecstasy has been demonized on both sides of the Atlantic, it will take a considerable effort to rehabilitate it as a safe and effective medicine, although it does seem to have genuine potential for therapeutic benefits.

Perhaps the last word should go to a patient, Melissa, a computer programmer in her mid-twenties being treated with ecstasy as part of psychotherapy for PTSD caused by abuse in childhood. Towards the end of the session Melissa said:

> Reliving this incident helped me free up my emotions in a number of ways. I know that I have a lot more to do, but I know now that I molded my views about the world–which I now know are not true–because that one incident caused me to distrust my parents . . . . I was able to dump my file–the medicine cleared my channels–insights and memories poured through me–fragments and pieces of the puzzle all came together. I had a cloud of trauma that had seemed in front of me–that for almost my whole life had been distorting my beliefs about myself–it seems behind me now, and I've gotten a new sense of who I am. (D. Adams and B. Fulton, *Salt Lake City Weekly*, 30 September 2004

CHAPTER 9

The future with amphetamines

'A Christmas package with a time bomb inside'
(Grinspoon and Hedblom 1975)

9.1. Introduction

Previous chapters have reviewed the various uses and abuses of amphetamines in our societies. These man-made chemicals had a great impact on life in the twentieth century and seem set to continue as major players—for good as well as evil. This concluding review will attempt to put some perspective on the use and abuse of these drugs and attempt some predictions of future trends.

9.2. Medical uses of amphetamines

The principal medical use of amphetamines will continue to be in treating ADHD. Despite the controversies that have raged around this subject, the scientific evidence that amphetamines can benefit many children with ADHD is convincing. Alleviating the often disturbing symptoms of the condition can benefit not only the children themselves, but also parents and siblings who may suffer distress and disruption to normal family life. However, there will continue to be controversy about where to draw the line. Are amphetamines suitable treatment for up to 10 per cent of all school children as some in the USA would argue, or is the UK target of treating 1 per cent of the most severely affected the more correct figure? The use of amphetamines to treat an adult form of ADHD is very new and likely to expand, but here too there will need to be clearer definition of who can really benefit from such treatment. As always, the pharmaceutical companies will exert subtle and not so subtle marketing pressure to increase the sales of their amphetamine-based products. In terms of pharmaceutical innovation, the older formulations of these drugs, which could easily be misused by injection or insufflation, will be replaced by sustained-release formulations. These involve incorporating the drug into a resin or other matrix which does not permit extraction of the active drug. Another idea being pursued by the UK company Shire Pharmaceuticals is to conjugate amphetamine chemically to an amino acid to form a 'pro-drug'. This could only release active amphetamine after digestion in the gut, thus precluding use by any route other than the oral one for which the drug is intended. As emphasized many times before, it is when amphetamines are taken by routes which permit rapid delivery to the brain that they are most dangerous and addictive.

The remaining medical uses are relatively small and are likely to diminish still further. The amphetamines have little long-term benefit in the treatment of obesity, although a number of amphetamine-based products remain on the market on both sides of the Atlantic. The fact they this is so has more to do with the lobbying power of the pharmaceutical industry than genuine medical need, and eventually these products will be phased out because of their unfavourable risk–benefit ratios. Similarly, the use of amphetamines in the treatment of narcolepsy, although based on genuine medical evidence, is likely to diminish as safer non-scheduled medicines such as modafinil take over.

The intriguing question of whether ecstasy will at last find proper medical uses remains open. As reviewed in the previous chapter, in the 1950s and 1960s many American psychiatrists and psychoanalysts were enthusiastic about the use of ecstasy, and there remains strong support from some sectors for the reinstatement of ecstasy in the treatment of certain psychiatric conditions, notably post-traumatic stress disorder. If the clinical trials that are now in progress yield positive results, there will be strong pressure for permitting a limited use of ecstasy in psychiatric medicine.

9.3. The continuing spread of illicit amphetamine abuse

The current epidemic of methamphetamine abuse in the USA and Southeast Asia shows little sign of abating. However, previous epidemics have come and gone, and perhaps this one will also wane in due course. Although the ability of methamphetamine to cause long-term damage to the brain has almost certainly been exaggerated, there is no doubt that heavy chronic use of the drug can cause serious personal and social damage, and it is hard to curb the spread of a drug that is so easy to manufacture illegally. In the Western world we can only hope that increasingly severe restrictions on the availability of the precursor and other chemicals needed for methamphetamine manufacture, together with a possible reclassification of the drug to the highest level of dangerous narcotic, may help to slow down the epidemic. In Southeast Asia some means must be found to curb the activities of the illegal Wa Army, and to persuade China and other countries in the region to place more restrictions on the availability of ephedrine and other chemicals needed for illicit manufacture.

By the beginning of the twenty-first century the popularity of ecstasy had waned somewhat, with reports of a 20 per cent decline in the numbers of people regularly using the drug in the UK. Nevertheless, it remains hugely popular, with approximately half a million users in the UK each weekend and 8 million worldwide. Meanwhile methamphetamine has also increased in popularity, sometimes replacing ecstasy in rave dance culture events. Current trends suggest that ecstasy may have passed its peak of popularity among teenagers and young adults on both sides of the Atlantic. According to the US Department of Health and Human Services *2003 National Survey on Drug Use and Health*, the number of past-year users was down from 3.2 million in 2002 to 2.1 million in 2003. Ecstasy is not so cool any more—it has lost some of its panache. In the USA a combination of more successful controls over imports of the drug, higher prices, and increasing recognition by young people of the safety messages given out by the government have combined to produce a decline in ecstasy use for the first time for many years—a rare example, perhaps, that government drug policy can sometimes be effective.

9.4. How can we treat amphetamine addiction?

9.4.1. Acute overdose

There is no single antagonist drug that can be used in emergency to block all the adverse effects of amphetamine overdose. However, efforts can be made to reduce the damaging hyperthermia, and β-blockers and other antihypertensive drugs can be used to counteract high blood pressure and overstimulation of the heart. The antipsychotic drug haloperidol is effective in blocking the psychostimulant effects of the drug that can lead to combative and violent behaviour (Murray 1998; Malay 2001).

9.4.2. Withdrawal, craving, and relapse

Withdrawal from amphetamine or methamphetamine is characterized by a protracted period of depression and unhappiness, usually accompanied by intense urges to use the drug. These urges can be prompted particularly strongly by conditioned cues in the user's environment previously associated with drug-taking (people, places, or objects).

There are few, if any, effective medicines that can counteract these strong and unpleasant symptoms. Several attempts have been made to use antidepressant drugs (fluoxetine, imipramine, desipramine, amlodipine), but, although fluoxetine may help initially to reduce craving, no long-term reduction in amphetamine use or other benefits have been seen seen (Srisurapanont *et al.* 2003). In local areas of England substitute prescribing of amphetamine has been attempted. This involves giving orally administered amphetamine to addicts who habitually inject the drug. The justification was to encourage amphetamine users into treatment so that their drug intake can be stabilized, to reduce their injecting behaviour and the accompanying health risks of street amphetamine, to reduce the risk of HIV and other viral infections, and to expose the addicts to education and psychosocial therapy. Descriptive results suggested an overall improvement in treated patients (Lingford-Hughes *et al.* 2004), but the results of a randomized controlled trial in Australia failed to show any significant benefits from amphetamine substitution plus counselling versus counselling alone (Shearer *et al.* 2001).

Psychosocial counselling remains the mainstay for the treatment of amphetamine addiction. In California an intensive outpatient therapeutic programme for cocaine and methamphetamine dependence called the 'Matrix model' has been developed (Rawson *et al.* 1995; Huber *et al.* 1997). The programme involves highly structured interviews over a period of 16–26 weeks, with up to 56 individual sessions covering drug education, relapse prevention, family involvement, and self-help, accompanied by regular drug testing. A study involving 500 methamphetamine-dependent subjects on the Matrix model indicated a considerable reduction in drug-positive urine tests (Huber *et al.* 1997). In a further controlled trial in which subjects were randomly assigned to the Matrix model or a standard outpatient treatment programme, the Matrix regime proved more effective in persuading subjects to stay with the treatment and providing longer periods of drug abstinence (Rawson *et al.* 2000, 2004). There is room for much improvement. Psychosocial counselling is expensive and requires well-trained staff. On both sides of the Atlantic resources and facilities for treating amphetamine addiction remain far too small to meet the growing need.

9.5. New problems for the future

Amphetamines are not going to go away. Most of the millions who regularly use these drugs will continue to do so, and a majority of these have learned to live with the drug without serious harm. Many use the drugs orally in a sporadic manner according to need. However, the increasingly widespread use of the drugs makes their control ever more difficult. In the use of amphetamines to treat ADHD we already see the difficulty of restricting their use. With so many young people now treated with amphetamines, it is already difficult to prevent their diversion to non-medical uses.

In sports there will always be some participants who seek to outwit the system and continue to use amphetamines or related drugs to improve performance. Children or students with ADHD can already obtain special dispensation to use amphetamine even when participating in sports events. Does this give them an unfair advantage?

Finally, although the Shulgins may have reached the end of their own personal chemical pilgrimage, many further chemical modifications of the basic amphetamine molecule remain to be explored. Who knows when another 'ecstasy' may be found, perhaps combining some unique permutation of dopamine, norepinephrine, and serotonin-boosting potential that will confer a new psychopharmacological profile? A pill to keep you awake for the entire weekend without hangover? Or one that confers happiness and empathy without any of the risks of ecstasy?

References

Abenhaim L, Moride Y, Brenot F, *et al.* (1996) Appetite suppressant drugs and the risk of primary pulmonary hypertension. *N Engl J Med*, **335**, 609–616.

Abi-Dargham A, Gil R, Krystal J, *et al.* (1998) Increased striatal dopamine transmission in schizophrenia: confirmation in a second cohort. *Am J Psychiatry*, **155**, 761–767.

Abi-Dargham A, Rodenhiser J, Printz D, *et al.* (2000) Increased baseline occupancy of D_2 receptors by dopamine in schizophrenia. *Proc Natl Acad Sci USA*, **97**, 8104–8109.

Adlersberg D, Mayer ME (1949) Results of prolonged medical treatment of obesity with diet alone, diet and thyroid preparations, and diet and amphetamine. *J Clin Endocrinol*, **9**, 275–284.

Albers DS, Sonsalla PK (1995) Methamphetamine-induced hyperthermia and dopaminergic neurotoxicity in mice: pharmacological profile of protective and neuroprotective agents. *J Pharmacol Exp Ther*, **275**, 1104–1114.

Alles GA (1928) The comparative physiological action of phenylethanolamine. *J Pharmacol Exp Ther*, **32**, 121–133.

Altschule MD, Iglauer A (1940) The effect of Benzedrine (β-phenylisopropylamine sulphate) and paredrine (p-hydroxy-α-methyl-phenylethylamine hydrobromide) on the circulation, metabolism and respiration in normal man. *J Clin Invest*, **19**, 497–502.

American Medical Association–Council on Pharmacy and Chemistry (1937) Present status of Benzedrine sulfate. *JAMA*, **109**, 2064–2069.

American Medical Association–Council on Drugs (1963) New drugs and development in therapeutics. *JAMA*, **183**, 362–363.

American Psychiatric Association (2000) *Diagnostic and Statistical Manual of Mental Disorders* (4th edn, Text Revision) (DSM-IV-TR). Washington, DC: American Psychiatric Association.

Angrist B (1994) Amphetamine psychosis: clinical variations of the syndrome. Cho AK, Segal DS (ed) *Amphetamine and its Analogs: Neuropharmacology, Toxicology and Abuse*. New York: Academic Press, 387–414.

Angrist B, Gershon S (1969) Amphetamine abuse in New York City—1966 to 1968. *Semin Psychiatry*, **1**, 195–207.

Angrist B, Gershon S (1970) The phenomenology of experimentally induced amphetamine psychosis. *Biol Psychiatry*, **2**, 95–107.

Angrist B, Sudilovsky A (1978) Central nervous system stimulants: historical aspects and clinical effects. In: Iversen LL, Iversen SD, Snyder SH (ed) *Handbook of Psychopharmacology*, Vol 11. New York: Plenum Press, 99–165.

Angrist B, Schweitzer JW, Gershon A, Friedhoff AJ (1970) Mephentermine psychosis: misuse of the Wyamine inhaler. *Am J Psychiatry*, **126**, 149–151.

Angrist B, Lee HK, Gershon S (1974) The antagonism of amphetamine-induced symptomatology by a neuroleptic. *Am J Psychiatry*, **131**, 817–819.

Angrist B, Rotrosen J, Gershon S (1980a) Response to apomorphine, amphetamine and neuroleptics in schizophrenic subjects. *Psychopharmacology*, **67**, 31–38.

Angrist B, Rotrosen J, Gershon S (1980b) Differential effects of amphetamine and neuroleptics on negative v positive symptoms in schizophrenia. *Psychopharmacology*, **72**, 17–19.

Angrist B, Rotrosen J, Gershon S (2001) Commentary on 'Differential effects of amphetamine and neuroleptics on negative v positive symptoms in schizophrenia', *Psychopharmacology* (1980), 72: 17–19. *Psychopharmacology*, **158**, 219–221.

Arnfred T, Randrup A (1968) Cholinergic mechanisms in brain inhibiting amphetamine-induced stereotyped behavior. *Acta Pharmacol Toxicol*, **26**, 384–394.

Arnold LE (2000) Methylphenidate versus amphetamine: a comparative review. In: Greenhill LL, Osman BB (ed) *Ritalin, Theory and Practice*. New Rochelle, NY: Mary Ann Liebert, 127–139.

Arnold LE, Wender PH, Snyder SH (1972) Levoamphetamine and dextroamphetamine: comparative efficacy in the hyperkinetic syndrome. *Arch Gen Psychiatry*, **27**, 816–822.

Arterburn DE, Crane PK, Veenstra DL (2004) The efficacy and safety of Sibutramine for weight loss: a systematic review. *Arch Intern Med*, **164**, 994–1003.

Bahnsen P, Jacobsen E, Thesleff H (1938) The subjective effects of beta-phenylisopropylaminsulfate on normal adults. *Acta Med Scand*, **97**, 89–131.

Balster RL, Schuster CR (1973) A comparison of D-amphetamine, L-amphetamine and methamphetamine self-administration in rhesus monkeys. *Pharmacol Biochem Behav*, **1**, 67–71.

Banerjee D, Vitiello MV, Grunstein RR (2004) Pharmacotherapy for excessive daytime sleepiness. *Sleep Med Rev*, **8**, 339–354.

Bell DS (1973) The experimental induction of amphetamine psychosis. *Arch Gen Psychiatry*, **29**, 35–40.

Bellarosa A, Bedford JA, Wilson MC (1980) Sociopharmacology of D-amphetamine in *Macaca arctoides*. *Pharmacol Biochem Behav*, **13**, 221–228.

Berridge KC, Robinson TE (1998) What is the role of dopamine in reward: hedonic impact, reward learning or incentive salience? *Brain Res Rev*, **28**, 309–369.

Bett WR (1946) Benzedrine sulphate in clinical medicine: a survey of the literature. *Postgrad Med J*, **22**, 205–218.

Bett WR, Howells LH, Macdonald AD (1955) *Amphetamine in Clinical Medicine: Actions and Uses*. Edinburgh: Livingstone.

Bhagat B, Wheeler N (1973) Effect of amphetamine on the swimming endurance of rats. *Neuropharmacology*, **12**, 711–713.

Bird ED, Spokes EG, Iversen LL (1979) Increased dopamine concentration in limbic areas of brain from patients dying with schizophrenia. *Brain*, **102**, 347–360.

Bobb AJ, Castellanos FX, Addington AM, Rapoport JL (2005) Molecular genetic studies of attention deficit hyperactivity disorder 1991–2004. *Am J Med Genet B Neuropsychiatr Genet*, **132**, 109–125.

Bower EA (2003) Use of amphetamines in the military environment. *Lancet*, **362** (Suppl), 18–19.

Bowyer JF, Davies DL, Schmued L, *et al.* (1994) Further studies of the role of hyperthermia in methamphetamine neurotoxicity. *J Pharmacol Exp Ther*, **268**, 1571–1580.

Bradley C (1937) The behavior of children receiving Benzedrine. *Am J Psychiatry*, **94**, 577–585.

Bradley C, Bowen M (1941) Amphetamine (Benzedrine) therapy of children's behavior disorders. *Am J Orthopsychiatry*, **11**, 92–103.

Brauer LH, Goudie AJ, de Wit H (1997) Dopamine ligands and the stimulus effects of amphetamine: animal models versus human laboratory data. *Psychopharmacology*, **130**, 2–13.

Breese GR, Cooper BR, Mueller RA (1974) Evidence for involvement of 5-hydroxytryptamine in the actions of amphetamine. *Br J Pharmacol*, **52**, 307–314.

Breier A, Su TP, Saunders R, *et al.* (1997) Schizophrenia is associated with elevated amphetamine-induced synaptic dopamine concentrations: evidence from a novel positron emission tomography method. *Proc Natl Acad Sci USA*, **94**, 2569–2574.

BMJ (1939) Editorial: Benzedrine, *BMJ*, **ii**, 25.

Brody AL, Mandelkern MA, Jarvik ME, *et al.* (2004) Differences between smokers and non-smokers in regional gray matter volumes and densities. *Biol Psychiatry*, **55**, 77–84.

Bronstein DM, Hong J-S (1995) Effects of sulpiride and SCH 23390 on methamphetamine-induced changes in body temperature and lethality. *J Pharmacol Exp Ther*, **274**, 943–950.

Buchert R, Thomasius R, Wilke F, *et al.* (2004) A voxel-based PET investigation of the long term effects of 'Ecstasy' consumption on brain serotonin transporters. *Am J Psychiatry*, **161**, 1181–1189.

Burt DR, Creese I, Snyder SH (1977) Antischizophrenic drugs: chronic treatment elevates dopamine receptor binding in brain. *Science*, **196**, 326–328.

Cadet JL, Jayanthi S, Deng X (2003) Speed kills: cellular and molecular bases of methamphetamine-induced nerve terminal degeneration and neuronal apoptosis. *FASEB J*, **17**, 1775–1788.

Cantwell R (2000) Commentary. *Adv Psychiatr Treat*, **6**, 39–40.

Carey JT, Mandel J (1968) A San Francisco Bay Area 'speed' scene. *J Health Soc Behav*, **9**, 164–174.

Carey JT, Mandel J (1969) The Bay Area 'speed' scene. *J Psychedelic Drugs*, **2**, 189–209.

Carlsson A, Lindqvist J (1963) Effect of chlorpromazine and haloperidol on formation of 3-methoxytyramine and normetanephrine in mouse brain. *Acta Pharmacol Toxicol*, **20**, 140–144.

Carlton PL (1968) Cholinergic mechanism in the control of behavior. In: Efron DH (ed) *Psychopharmacology: A Review of Progress*. Washington, DC: US Government Printing Office, 123–135.

Cass WA, Manning MW (1999) Recovery of presynaptic dopaminergic functioning in rats treated with neurotoxic doses of methamphetamine. *J Neurosci*, **19**, 7653–7660.

Chan YP, Swanson JM, Soldin SS, Thiessen JJ, Macleod SM, Logan W (1983) Methylphenidate hydrochloride given with or before breakfast. II: Effects on plasma concentration of methylphenidate and ritalinic acid. *Pediatrics*, **72**, 56–59.

Chance MRA (1946) Aggregation as a factor influencing the toxicity of sympathomimetic amines in mice. *J Pharmacol*, **87**, 214–219.

Chang L, Ernst T, Speck O, *et al.* (2002) Perfusion MRI and computerized cognitive test abnormalities in abstinent methamphetamine users. *Psychiatry Res*, **114**, 65–79.

Check E (2004) The ups and downs of ecstasy. *Nature*, **429**, 126–128.

Chiueh CC, Moore KE (1976) Dopaminergic agonists and electrical stimulation of the midbrain raphé on the release of 5-hydroxytryptamine from the cat brain *in vivo*. *J Neurochem*, **26**, 319–324.

Cho AK (1990) Ice: a new dosage form of an old drug. *Science*, **249**, 631–634.

Cho AK, Melega WP, Kuczenski R, Segal DS (2001) Relevance of pharmacokinetic parameters in animal models of methamphetamine abuse. *Synapse*, **39**, 161–166.

Choury PA, Meissonnier J (2004) *Yaa Baa: Production, Traffic and Consumption of Methamphetamines in Mainland and Southeast Asia*. Singapore: Singapore University Press.

Clement-Cormier YC, Kebabian JW, Petzold GL, Greengard P (1974) Dopamine-sensitive adenylate cyclase in mammalian brain: a possible site of action of antipsychotic drugs. *Proc Natl Acad Sci USA*, **71**, 1113–1117.

Cole JC, Bailey M, Sumnall HR, Wagstaff GF, King LA (2002) The content of ecstasy tablets: implications for the study of their long term-effects. *Addiction*, **97**, 1531–1536.

Colman E (2004) FDA regulation of obesity drugs 1938–1999. *FDA Endocrinology and Metabolic Drugs Advisory Committee*, 8 September 2004.

Condon J, Smith N (2003) Prevalence of drug use: key findings from the 2002/03 British Crime Survey. *Home Office Research Study 229*. London: Home Office.

Connell PH (1958) *Amphetamine Psychosis*. London: Oxford University Press.

Conners CK (1969) A teachers' rating scale for use in drug studies with children. *Am J Psychiatry*, **126**, 884–888.

Conners CK (1998) Rating scales in attention deficit hyperactivity disorder: use in assessment and treatment monitoring. *J Clin Psychiatry*, **59** (Suppl 7), 24–30.

Conners CK, Sitarenios G, Parker JD, Epstein JN (1998) Revision and standardization of the Conners Teacher Rating Scale (CTRS-R): factor structure, reliability, and criterion validity. *J Abnorm Child Psychol*, **26**, 279–291.

Connolly HM, Crary JL, McGoon MD, *et al.* (1997) Valvular heart disease associated with fenfluramine–phentermine. *N Engl J Med*, **337**, 581–588.

Corkery JM (2002) *Drug Seizure and Offender Statistics 2000—United Kingdom*. London: Home Office.

Costa E, Groppetti A, Naimzada MK (1972) Effects of amphetamine on the turnover rate of brain catecholamines and motor activity. *Br J Pharmacol*, **44**, 742–751.

Creese I, Iversen SD (1974) The role of forebrain dopamine systems in amphetamine induced stereotypy in the adult rat following neonatal treatment with 6-hydroxydopamine. *Psychopharmacology*, **39**, 345–357.

Creese I, Burt DR, Snyder SH (1976a) Dopamine receptor binding predicts clinical and pharmacological potencies of antischizophrenic drugs. Science, **192**, 481–483.

Creese I, Burt DR, Snyder SH (1976b) Dopamine receptors and average clinical doses. *Science*, **194**, 546.

Cross AJ, Crow TJ, Owen F (1981) ^{3}H-Flupenthixol binding in post-mortem brains of schizophrenics: evidence for a selective increase in dopamine D_2 receptors. *Psychopharmacology*, **74**, 122–124.

Crow TJ (1980) Molecular pathology of schizophrenia: more than one disease process? *Br Med J*, **280**, 66–68.

Curran C, Byrappa N, McBride A (2004) Stimulant psychosis: systematic review. *Br J Psychiatry*, **185**, 196–204.

Curzon G, Gibson EL (1999) The serotonergic appetite suppressant fenfluramine: reappraisal and rejection. In: Huerther G, Kochen W, Simat TJ, Steinhart H (ed) *Tryptophan, Serotonin and Melatonin: Basic Aspects and Applications*. New York: Kluwer Academic–Plenum, 95–100.

Curzon G, Gibson EL, Oluyomi AO (1997) Appetite suppression by commonly used drugs depends on 5-HT receptors but not 5-HT availability. *Trends Pharmac Sci*, **18**, 21–25.

Cuthbertson DP, Knox JAC (1947) The effects of analeptics on the fatigued subject. *J Physiol*, **106**, 42–58.

Davidson C, Gow AJ, Lee TH, Ellinwood EH (2001) Methamphetamine neurotoxicity: necrotic and apoptotic mechanisms and relevance to human abuse and treatment. *Brain Res Rev*, **36**, 1–22.

Davis KL, Kahn RS, Ko G, Davidson M (1991) Dopamine and schizophrenia: a review and reconceptualization. *Am J Psychiatry*, **148**, 1474–1486.

Davison D, Parrott AC (1997) Ecstasy in recreational users: self-reported psychological and physiological effects. *Hum Psychopharmacol*, **12**, 91–97.

de la Torre R, Farré M (2004) Neurotoxicity of MDMA (ecstasy): the limitations of scaling from animals to humans. *Trends Pharmacol Sci*, **25**, 505–508.

Delay J, Deniker T, Harl JM (1952) Utilisation en thérapeutique psychiatrique d'une phénothiazine d'action centrale selective (4560 RP). *Ann Med Psychol (Paris)*, **110**, 112–117.

Denney CB, Rapport MD (2001) Cognitive pharmacology of stimulants in children with ADHD. In: Solanto MV, Arnsetein AFT, Castellanos FX (ed) *Stimulant Drugs and ADHD*. Oxford: Oxford University Press, 283–302.

Dews PB, Winger GR (1977) Rate-dependency of the behavioral effects of amphetamine. In: Thompson T, Dews PB (ed) *Advances in Behavioral Pharmacology*, Vol. 1. New York: Academic Press, 167–227.

Diaz-Veliz G, Baeza R, Benavente F, Dussaubat N, Mora S (1994) Influence of the oestrus cycle and oestradiol on the behavoural effects of amphetamine and apomorphine in rats. *Pharmacol Biochem Behav*, 49, 819–825.

Di Chiara G, Bassareo V, Fenu S, *et al.* (2004) Dopamine and drug addiction: the nucleus accumbens shell connection. *Neuropharmacology*, 47, 227–241.

Ding YS, Gatley SJ, Thanos PK, *et al.* (2004) Brain kinetics of methylphenidate (Ritalin) enantiomers after oral administration. *Synapse*, 53, 168–175.

Dowling GP, McDonough E, Bost R (1987) 'Eve' and 'Ecstasy'. A report of five deaths associated with the use of MDEA and MDMA. *JAMA*, 257, 1615–1617.

Duvauchelle CL, Levitin M, MacConell LA, Lee LK, Ettenberg A (1992) Opposite effects of prefrontal cortex and nucleus accumbens infusions of flupenthixol on stimulant-induced locomotion and brain stimulation reward. *Brain Res*, 576, 104–110.

Eisner B (1989) *Ecstasy: the MDMA Story*. Berkeley, CA: Ronin Press.

Ellinwood EH Jr (1967) Amphetamine psychosis: description of the individuals and the process. *J Nerv Ment Dis*, 144, 273–283.

Ellinwood EH Jr (1969) Amphetamine psychosis: a multi-dimensional process. *Semin Psychiatry*, 1, 208–226.

Ellinwood EH Jr (1971) Assault and homicide associated with amphetamine abuse. *Am J Psychiatry*, 127, 1170–1175.

Ellinwood EH Jr (1972) Amphetamine psychosis: individuals, settings and sequences. In: Ellinwood EH, Cohen S (ed) *Current Concepts on Amphetamine Abuse*. Washington, DC: US Government Printing Office, 143–157.

Estaban B, O'Shea E, Camarero J, Sanchez V, Green AR, Colado MI (2001) 3,4-Methylenedioxymethamphetamine induces monoamine release, but not toxicity, when administered centrally at a concentration occurring following a peripherally injected neurotoxic dose. *Psychopharmacology*, 154, 251–260.

Everitt BJ, Dickinson A, Robbins TW (2001) The neuropsychological basis of addictive behaviour. *Brain Res Brain Res Rev*, 36, 129–138.

Fantegrossi WE, Woolverton WL, Kilbourn M, *et al.* (2004) Behavioral and neurochemical consequences of long term intravenous self-administration of MDMA and its enantiomers by rhesus monkeys. *Neuropsychopharmacology*, 29, 1270–1281.

Faraone SV, Biederman J (1998) Neurobiology of attention-deficit hyperactivity disorder. *Biol Psychiatry*, 44, 951–958.

Faraone SV, Biederman J, Roe C (2002) Comparative efficacy of Adderall and methylphenidate in attention deficity hyperactivity disorder: a meta-analysis. *J Clin Psychopharmacol*, **22**, 468–473.

Faraone SV, Spencer T, Aleardi M, Pagano C, Biederman J (2004) Meta-analysis of the efficacy of methylphenidate for treating adult attention deficit/ hyperactivity disorder. *J Clin Psychopharmacol*, **24**, 24–29.

Farde L, Wiesel FA, Stone-Elander S, *et al.* (1990) D_2 dopamine receptors in neuroleptic-naive schizophrenic patients. A positron emission tomography study with [^{11}C]-raclopride. *Arch Gen Psychiatry*, **47**, 213–219.

Ferraro L, Antonelli T, O'Connor WT, Tanganelli S, Rambert FA, Fuxe K (1997) Modafinil: an antinarcoleptic drug with a different neurochemical profile to D-amphetamine and dopamine uptake blockers. *Biol Psychiatry*, **42**, 1181–1183.

Ferris RM, Tang FLM, Maxwell RA (1972) A comparison of the capacities of isomers of amphetamine, deoxypipradol and methylphenidate to inhibit the uptake of tritiated catecholamines into rat cerebral cortex slices, synaptosomal preparations of rat cerebral cortex, hypothalamus and striatum and into adrenergic nerves of rabbit aorta. *J Pharmacol Exp Ther*, **181**, 407–416.

Finch JW (1947) The overweight obstetric patient with special reference to the use of Dexedrine sulfate. *J Okla State Med Assoc*, **40**,119–122.

Fisher E, Fisher D (2003) *Been There Done That*. New York: Thomas Dunne.

Fishman AP (1999) Aminorex to fen/phen. *Circulation* **99**, 156–161.

Fitzgerald LW, Burn TC, Brown BS, *et al.* (2000) Possible role of valvular serotonin 5-HT(2B) receptors in the cardiopathy associated with fenfluramine. *Mol Pharmacol*, **57**, 75–81.

Fleckenstein AE, Gibb JW, Hanson GR (2000) Differential effects of stimulants on monoaminergic transporters: pharmacological consequences and implications for neurotoxicity. *Eur J Pharmacol*, **406**, 1–13.

Follath F, Burkhart F and Schweizer W (1971) Drug-induced pulmonary hypertension? *BMJ*, **i**, 265–266.

Freed SC, Hays EE (1959) A new nonamphetamine anorectic agent. *Am J Med Sci*, **238**, 55–59.

Frosch D, Shoptaw S, Huber A, Rawson RA, Ling W (1996) Sexual HIV risk among gay and bisexual male methamphetamine abusers. *J Subst Abuse Treat*, **13**, 483–486.

Fukui S, Wada K, Iyo M (1994) Epidemiology of amphetamine abuse in Japan and its social implications. In: Cho AK, Segal DS (ed) *Amphetamine and its Analogs: Neuropharmacology, Toxicology and Abuse*. New York: Academic Press, 459–479.

Gatley SJ, Pan DF, Chen R, Chaturvedi G, Ding YS (1996) Affinities of methylphenidate derivatives for dopamine, norepinephrine and serotonin transporters. *Life Sci*, **58**, 231–239.

Gearing J (1999) Thailand's battle for its soul. *Asiaweek*, 13 August 1999.

Gelvin EP, McGavack TH (1949) Dexedrine and weight reduction. *NY State J Med*, **49**, 280–282.

Gerald MC (1978) Effects of (+)-amphetamine on the treadmill endurance performance of rats. *Neuropharmacology*, **17**, 703–704.

Gerra G, Zaimovic A, Giucastro G, *et al.* (1998) Serotonergic function after (±)3,4-methylenedioxymethamphetamine ('Ecstasy') in humans. *Int Clin Psychopharmacol*, **13**, 1–9.

Gibbs JW, Hanson GR, Johnson M (1996) Neurochemical mechanisms of toxicity. In: Cho AK, Segal DS (ed) *Amphetamine and its Analogs: Neuropharmacology, Toxicology and Abuse*. New York: Academic Press, 269–282.

Gill JR, Hayes JA, deSouza IS, Marken E, Stajic M (2002) Ecstasy (MDMA) deaths in New York City: a case series and review of the literature. *J Forensic Sci*, **47**, 121–126.

Gogos JA, Morgan M, Luine V, Santha M, Ogawa S, Pfaff D, Karayiorgou M (1998) Catechol-O-methyltransferase-deficient mice exhibit sexually dimorphic changes in catecholamine levels and behavior. *Proc Natl Acad Sci US*, **95**, 9991-9996.

Gordon CK, Watkinson WP, O'Callaghan JP, Miller DB (1991) Effects of 3,4-methylendioxymethamphetamine on autonomic thermoregulatory responses of the rat. *Pharmacol Biochem Behav*, **38**, 339–344.

Gottlieb JS (1949) The use of sodium amytal and Benzedrine sulfate in the symptomatic treatment of depressions. *Dis Nerv Syst*, **10**, 50–52.

Grace AA (2000) The tonic/phasic model of dopamine system regulation and its implications for understanding alcohol and psychostimulant craving. *Addiction*, **95** (Suppl 2), S119–S128.

Grace AA (2001) Psychostimulant actions on dopamine and limbic system function: relevance to the pathophysiology and treatment of ADHD. In: Solanto MV, Arnsetein AFT, Castellanos FX (ed) *Stimulant Drugs and ADHD*. Oxford: Oxford University Press, 134–157.

Graham DJ, Green L (1997) Further cases of valvular heart disease associated with fenfluramine–phentermine. *N Engl J Med*, **337**, 635.

Grahame-Smith DG (1971) Studies *in vivo* on the relationship between brain tryptophan, brain 5-HT synthesis and hyperactivity in rats treated with a monoamine oxidase inhibitor and L-tryptophan. *J Neurochem*, **18**, 1053–1066.

Green ER, Mechan AO, Elliott JM, O'Shea E, Colado I (2003) The pharmacology and clinical pharmacology of 3,4-methylenedioxymethamphetamine (MDMA, 'Ecstasy'). *Pharmacol Rev*, **55**, 463–508.

Greenberg HR, Lustig N (1966) Misuse of Dristan inhaler. *NY State J Med*, **66**, 613–617.

Griffith J, Oates JA, Cavanaugh JH (1968) Paranoid episodes induced by drug. *JAMA*, **205**, 39.

Griffith J, Davis J, Oates J (1971) Amphetamines: addiction to a non-addicting drug. *Pharmacopsychiatr Neuropsychopharmakol*, **4**, 60.

Grilly DM, Loveland A (2001) What is a 'low dose' of *d*-amphetamine for inducing behavioral effects? *Psychopharmacology*, **153**, 155–169.

Grinspoon L, Hedblom P (1975) *The Speed Culture. Amphetamine Use and Abuse in America*. Cambridge, MA: Harvard University Press.

Grob CS (2000) Deconstructing ecstasy: the politics of MDMA research. *Addict Res*, **8**, 549–588.

Gross MD (1976) A comparison of dextro-amphetamine and racemic amphetamine in the treatment of the hyperkinetic syndrome or minimal brain dysfunction. *Dis Nerv Syst*, **37**, 14–16.

Guilarte TR, Nihei MK, McGlothan JL, Howard AS (2003) Methamphetamine-induced deficits of brain monoaminergic neuronal markers: distal axotomy or neuronal plasticity. *Neuroscience*, **122**, 499–513.

Guix T, Hurd YL, Ungerstedt U (1992) Amphetamine enhances extracellular concentrations of dopamine and acetylcholine in dorsolateral striatum and nucleus accumbens of freely moving rats. *Neurosci Lett*, **138**, 137–140.

Gunne LM, Anggard E, Jönsson LE (1972) Clinical trials with amphetamine-blocking drugs. *Psychiatr Neurol Neurochir*, **75**, 225–226.

Gurtner HP (1985) Aminorex and pulmonary hypertension. *Cor Vasa*, **27**, 160–171.

Guttmann E (1936) The effect of Benzedrine on depressive states. *J Ment Sci*, **82**, 618–620.

Guttmann E, Sargant W (1937) Oservations on Benzedrine. *BMJ*, i, 1013–1015.

Halkitis PN, Parsons JT, Stiratt MJ (2001) A double epidemic: crystal methamphetamine drug use in relation to HIV transmission among gay men. *J Homosex*, **41**, 17–35.

Hanson GR, Rau KS, Fleckenstein AE (2004) The methamphetamine experience: a NIDA partnership. *Neuropharmacology*, **47**, 92–100.

Harris N (2005) *The History of Drugs: Amphetamines*. New York: Thomson Gale.

Harrison PJ, Owen MJ (2003) Genes for schizophrenia? Recent findings and their pathophysiological implications. *Lancet*, **361**, 417–419.

Hart CL, Ward AS, Haney M, Folin RW, Fischman MW (2001) Methamphetamine self-administration by humans. *Psychopharmacology*, **157**, 75–81.

Hatzidimitriou G, McCann UD, Ricaurte GA (1999) Altered serotonin innervation patterns in the forebrain of monkeys treated with (±)3,4-methylenedioxymethamphetamine seven years previously: factors influencing abnormal recovery. *J Neurosci*, **19**, 5096–5107.

Hechtman L, Greenfield B (2003) Long-term use of stimulants in children with attention deficit hyperactivity disorder: safety, efficacy, and long-term outcome. *Paediatr Drugs*, **5**, 787–794.

Heinz A, Jones DW (2000) Serotonin transporters in ecstasy users. *Br J Psychiatr*, **176**, 193–194.

Hemmi T (1969) How we handled the problem of drug abuse in Japan. In: Sjöqvist F, Tottie M (ed) *Abuse of Central Stimulants*. Stockholm: Almqvist and Wiksell, 147–153.

Herman M, Nagler SH (1954) Psychoses due to amphetamine. *J Nerv Ment Dis*, **120**, 268–272.

Heston LL, Heston R (1979) *The Medical Casebook of Adolf Hitler*. New York: Cooper Square Press.

Heyrodt H, Weissenstein H (1940) Über Steigerung korperlicher Leistungfahigkeit durch Pervitin. *Naunyn Schmiedebergs Arch Exp Pathol Pharmakol*, **195**, 273–275.

Hoebel BG (1977) The psychopharmacology of feeding. In: Iversen LL, Iversen SD, Snyder SH (ed) *Handbook of Psychopharmacology*, Vol 8. New York: Plenum Press, 55–130.

Holland J (2001a) The history of MDMA. In: Holland J (ed) *Ecstasy: The Complete Guide*. Rochester, VT: Park Street Press, 11–20.

Holland J (ed) (2001b) *Ecstasy: The Complete Guide*. Rochester, VT: Park Street Press.

Hollister AS, Breese GR, Cooper BR (1974) Comparison of tyrosine hydroxylase and dopamine-β-hydroxylase inhibition with the effects of various 6-hydroxydopamine treatments on *d*-amphetamine-induced motor activity. *Psychopharmacology*, **36**, 1–16.

Huber A, Ling W, Shoptaw S, Gulati V, Brethen P, Rawson, R. (1997) Integrating treatments for methamphetamine abuse: a psychosocial perspective. *J Addict Dis* **16**, 41–50.

Hurd YL, Ungerstedt U (1989) *In vivo* neurochemical profile of dopamine uptake inhibitors and releasers in rat caudate-putamen. *Eur J Pharmacol*, **166**, 251–260.

Independent Drug Monitoring Unit (2004) Amphetamine and sex. Available online at: http://www.idmu.co.uk/amphetsex.htm

Israel JA, Lee K (2002) Amphetamine usage and genital self-mutilation. *Addiction*, **97**, 1215–1218.

Iversen LL (2001) *A Very Short Introduction to Drugs*. Oxford: Oxford University Press.

Iversen LL, Mackay AV (1981) Brain dopamine receptor densities in schizophrenia. *Lancet*, **ii**, 149

Janowsky JS, El-Yousef KK, Davis JM, Sekerke HJ (1973) Provocation of schizophrenic symptoms by intravenous-administration of methylphenidate. *Arch Gen Psychiatry*, **28**, 185–191.

JAMA (1937) Editorial: Benzedrine sulfate 'pep pills'. *JAMA*, **108**, 1973–1974.

Janssen PAG, Niemegeers CJE, Schellekens JHL (1965) Is it possible to predict the clinical effects of neuroleptic drugs (major tranquilizers) from animal data? Part I: Neuroleptic activity spectra for rats. *Arzneimittelforschung*, **15**, 104–117.

Johanson CE, Balster RL, Bonese K (1976) Self-administration of psychomotor stimulant drugs: the effects of unlimited access. *Pharmacol Biochem Behav*, **4**, 45–51.

Johnson BA, Ait-Daoud N, Wells LT (2000) Effects of isradipine, a dihydropyridine-class calcium channel antagonist, on *d*-methamphetamine-induced cognitive and physiological changes in humans. *Neuropsychopharmacology*, **22**, 504–512.

Jones AL, Simpson KJ (1999) Review article: mechanisms and management of hepatotoxicity in ecstasy (MDMA) and amphetamine intoxications. *Aliment Pharmacol Ther*, **13**, 129–133.

Jones SR, Gainetdinov RR, Wightman RM, Caron MG (1998) Mechanisms of amphetamine action revealed in mice lacking the dopamine transporter. *J Neurosci*, **18**, 1979–1986.

Jönsson LE (1972) Pharmacological blockade of amphetamine effects in amphetamine dependent subjects. *Eur J Clin Pharmacol*, **4**, 206–211.

Jönsson LE, Gunne LM, Angaard E (1969) Effects of alphamethyltyrosine in amphetamine dependent subjects. *Pharmacol Clin*, **2**, 27–29.

Jönsson LE, Angaard E, Gunne LM (1971) Blockade of intravenous amphetamine euphoria in man. *Clin Pharmacol Ther*, **12**, 889–896.

Kahlig KM, Binda F, Khoshbouei H, et al. (2005) Amphetamine induces dopamine efflux through a dopamine transporter channel. *Proc Natl Acad Sci USA*, **102**, 3495–3500.

Kalant H (2001) The pharmacology and toxicology of 'ecstasy' (MDMA) and related drugs. *Can Med Assoc J*, **165**, 917–928.

Kalant OJ (1973) *The Amphetamines: Toxicity and Addiction* (2nd edn). Springfield, IL: Charles C Thomas.

Kalix P (1992) Cathinone, a natural amphetamine. *Pharmacol Toxicol*, **70**, 77–86.

Kall K (1992) Effects of amphetamine on sexual behaviour of male i.v. drug users in Stockholm—a pilot study. *AIDS Educ Prev*, **4**, 6–17.

Kamien JB, Bickel WK, Hughes JR, Higgins ST, Smith BJ (1993) Drug discrimination by humans compared to nonhumans: current status and future directions. *Psychopharmacology*, **111**, 259–270.

Keating GM, Figgit DP (2002) Dexmethylphenidate. *Drugs*, **62**, 1899–1904.

Kebabian JW, Petzold GL, Greengard P (1972) Dopamine-sensitive adenylate cyclase in caudate nucleus of rat brain and its similarity to the 'dopamine receptor'. *Proc Natl Acad Sci USA*, **69**, 2145–2149.

Keitel W (1965) *The Memoirs of Field-Marshal Keitel*. New York: Stein and Day.

Kelly PH, Seviour PW, Iversen SD (1975) Amphetamine and apomorphine responses in the rat following 6-OHDA lesions of the nucleus accumbens septi and corpus striatum. *Brain Research*, **94**, 507–522.

Kenagy DN, Bird CT, Webber CM, Fischer JR (2004) Dextroamphetamine use during B-2 combat missions. *Aviat Space Environ Med*, **75**, 381–386.

Kiloh LG, Brandon S (1962) Habituation and addiction to amphetamines. *BMJ*, **ii**, 40–43.

Kinnell HG (2003) European withdrawal of appetite suppressants. *Obes Rev*, **4**, 79–81.

Kish SJ (2002) How strong is the evidence that brain serotonin neurons are damaged in human users of ecstasy? *Pharmacol Biochem Behav*, **71**, 845–855.

Kita T, Wagner GC, Nakashima T (2003) Current research on methamphetamine-induced neurotoxicity: animal models of monoamine disruption. *J Pharmacol Sci*, **92**, 178–195.

Klee H (1997a) Amphetamine misusers in contemporary Britain: the emergence of a hidden population. In: Klee H (ed) *Amphetamine Misuse*. Reading, UK: Harwood Academic, 19–34.

Klee H (1997b) A typology of amphetamine users in the United Kingdom. In: Klee H (ed) *Amphetamine Misuse*. Reading, UK: Harwood Academic, 35–68.

Klee H, Morris J (1994) Crime and drug misuse: economic and psychological aspects of the criminal activities of heroin and amphetamine injectors. *Addict Res*, **1**, 377–386.

Koch S, Galloway MP (1997) MDMA-induced dopamine release *in vivo*: role of endogenous serotonin. *J Neural Transm*, **104**, 135–146.

Koelega HS (1993) Stimulant drugs and vigilance performance: a review. *Psychopharmacology*, **111**, 1–16.

Koob GF, Sanna PP, Bloom FE (1998) Neuroscience of addiction. *Neuron*, **21**, 467–476.

Konuma, K (1994) Use and abuse of amphetamines in Japan. In: Cho AK, Segal DS (ed) *Amphetamine and its Analogs: Neuropharmacology, Toxicology and Abuse*. New York: Academic Press, 415–438.

Kornetsky C (1958) Effects of meprobamate, phenobarbital, and dextroamphetamine on reaction time and learning in man. *J Pharmacol Exp Ther*, **123**, 216–219.

Kornetsky C, Mirsky AF, Kessler EK, Dorff JE (1959) The effects of dextro-amphetamine on behavioral deficits produced by sleep loss in humans. *J Pharmacol Exp Ther*, **127**, 46–50.

Kramer JC (1969) Introduction to amphetamine abuse. *J Psychedelic Drugs*, **1**, 1–16.

Kramer JC (1972) Introduction to amphetamine abuse. In: Ellinwood EH, Cohen S (ed) *Current Concepts on Amphetamine Abuse*. Washington, DC: US Government Printing Office, 177–184.

Kramer JC, Vitezslav S, Fischman S, Littlefield DC (1967) Amphetamine abuse. *JAMA*, **201**, 89–93.

Kratofil PH, Baberg HT, Dimsdale JE (1996) Self-mutilation and severe self-injurious behavior associated with amphetamine psychosis. *Gen Hosp Psychiatry*, **18**, 117–120.

Kuczenski R, Segal DS (1992) Regional norepinephrine response to amphetamine using dialysis: comparison to caudate dopamine. *Synapse*, **11**, 164–169.

Kuczenski R, Segal DS (1997) Effects of methylphenidate on extracellular dopamine, serotonin and norepinephrine: comparison with amphetamine. *J Neurochem*, **68**, 2032–2037.

Laidler KAJ, Morgan P (1997) Kinship and community: the 'ice' crisis in Hawaii. In: Klee H (ed) *Amphetamine Misuse*. Reading, UK: Harwood Academic, 163–180.

Lake C, Quirk R (1984) Stimulants and look-alike drugs. *Psychiatr Clin North Am*, **7**, 689–701.

Lamb RJ, Henningfield JE (1994) Human *d*-amphetamine drug discrimination: methamphetamine and hydromorphine. *J Exp Anal Behav*, **61**, 169–180.

Lan KC, Lin YF, Yu FC, Lin CS, Chu P (1998) Clinical manifestations and prognostic features of acute methamphetamine intoxication. *J Formos Med Assoc*, **97**, 528–533.

Lancet (1971) Editorial. *Lancet*, **ii**, 252.

Landman M, Preisig R and Perlman M (1958) A practical mood stimulant. *J Med Soc NJ*, **55**, 55–58.

Larsen PJ, Vrang N, Tang-Christensen M, *et al.* (2002) Ups and downs for neuropeptides in body weight homeostasis: pharmacological potential of cocaine amphetamine regulated transcript and pre-proglucagon-derived peptides. *Eur J Pharmacol*, **440**, 159–172.

Laruelle M, Abi-Dargham A, van Dyk CH, *et al.* (1996) Single photon emission computerized tomography imaging of amphetamine-induced dopamine release in drug-free schizophrenic subjects. *Proc Natl Acad Sci USA*, **93**, 9235–9240.

Lasagna L (1973) Attitudes toward appetite suppressants: a survey of US physicians. *JAMA*, **225**, 44–48.

Lasagna L, von Felsinger JM, Beecher HK (1955) Drug-induced mood changes in man: I. Observations on healthy subjects, chronically ill patients and 'postaddicts'. *JAMA*, **157**, 1006–1020.

Laties VG, Weiss B (1981) The amphetamine margin in sports. *Fed Proc*, **40**, 2689–2692.

Leake CD (1958) *The Amphetamines: Their Actions and Uses*. Springfield IL: Charles C. Thomas, 123.

Lee T, Seeman P, Tourtelotte WW, Farley IJ, Hornykiewicz O (1978) Binding of ^{3}H-neuroleptics and ^{3}H-neuroleptics and ^{3}H-apomorphine in schizophrenic brains. *Nature*, **274**, 897–900.

Leonard BL, McCartan D, White J, King DJ (2004) Methylphenidate: a review of its neuropharmacological, neuropsychological and adverse clinical effects. *Hum Psychopharmacol*, **19**, 151–180.

Lesses MF, Myerson A (1938) Human autonomic pharmacology. XVI: Benzedrine sulfate (amphetamine) in obesity. *N Engl J Med*, **218**, 119–124.

Liang NY, Rutledge CO (1982) Comparison of the release of [3H]dopamine from isolated corpus striatum by amphetamine, fenfluramine and unlabelled dopamine. *Biochem Pharmacol*, **31**, 983–992.

Lingford-Hughes AR, Welch S, Nutt DJ (2004) Evidence-based guidelines for the pharmacological management of substance misuse, addiction and comorbidity: recommendations from the British Association for Psychopharmacology. *J Psychopharmacol*, **18**, 293–335.

Logan BK, Fligner CL, Haddix T (1998) Cause and manner of death in fatalities involving methamphetamine. *Am J Psychiatry*, **43**, 28–34.

Loke YK, Derry S, Pritchard-Copley A (2002) Appetite suppressants and valvular heart disease–a systematic review. *BMC Clin Pharmacol*, **2**, 6–16.

London ED, Simon SL, Berman SM, *et al.* (2004) Mood disturbances and regional cerebral metabolic abnormalities in recently abstinent methamphetamine abusers. *Arch Gen Psychiatry*, **61**, 73–84.

Lott DC, Kim SJ, Cook EH, de Wit, H (2005) Dopamine transporter gene associated with diminished subjective response to amphetamine. *Neuropsychopharmacology*, **30**, 602–609.

Mabry PD, Campbell BA (1973) Serotonergic inhibition of catecholamine-induced behavioral arousal. *Brain Res*, **49**, 381–391.

McCann UD, Ridenour A, Shaham Y, Ricaurte GA (1994) Brain serotoninergic neurotoxicity after MDMA ('Ecstasy'): a controlled study in humans. *Neuropsychopharmacology*, **10**, 129–138.

McCann UD, Seiden LS, Rubin LJ, Ricaurte GA (1997a) Brain serotonin neurotoxicity and primary pulmonary hypertension from fenfluramineand dexfenfluramine. *JAMA*, **278**, 666–672.

McCann UD, Mertl MM, Murphy DL, Post RP, Ricaurte GA (1997b) Neuroendocrine effects of intravenous metachlorophenylpiperazine in (±)3,4-methylenedioxymethamphetamine users. In: *American Psychiatric Association New Research Program and Abstracts*. Washington, DC: American Psychiatric Association, 147.

McCann UD, Yuan J, Ricaurte GA (1998a) Neurotoxic effects of (±)fenfluramine and phentermine, alone and in combination, on monoamine neurons in the mouse brain. *Synapse*, **30**, 239–246.

McCann UD, Szabo Z, Scheffel U, Dannals RF, Ricaurte GA (1998b) Positron emission tomographic evidence of toxic effects of MDMA ('Ecstasy') on brain serotonin neurons in human beings. *Lancet*, **352**, 1433–1437.

McCann UD, Wong DF, Yokoi F, Villemagne V, Dannals RF, Ricaurte GA (1998c) Reduced striatal dopamine transporter density in abstinent methamphetamine and methcathinone users: evidence from positron emission tomography studies with [^{11}C]WIN-35,428. *J Neurosci*, **18**, 8417–8422.

McCann UD, Eligulashvili V, Ricaurte GA (2000) (±)3,4-Methylene-dioxymethamphetamine ('Ecstasy')-induced serotonin neurotoxicity: clinical studies. *Neuropsychobiology*, **42**, 11–16.

McGough JJ, Barkley RA (2004) Diagnostic controversies in adult attention deficit/hyperactivity disorder. *Am J Psychiatry*, **161**, 1948–1956.

McGough JJ, Biederman J, Greenhill JJ, *et al.* (2003) Pharmacokinetics of SL1381 (Adderall XR), an extended-release formulation of Adderall. *J Am Acad Child Adolesc Psychiatry*, **42**, 684–691.

McGowan S, Lawrence AD, Sales T, Quested D, Grasby P (2004) Presynaptic dopaminergic dysfunction in schizophrenia. *Arch Gen Psychiatry*, **61**, 134–142.

McGuire P (2000) Long term psychiatric and cognitive effects of MDMA use. *Toxicol Lett*, **112–113**, 153–156.

Mackay AVP, Bird ED, Spokes EG, *et al.* (1980) Dopamine receptors and schizophrenia: drug effect or illness? *Lancet*, **ii**, 915–916.

McKetin R, Mattick RP (1997) Attention and memory in illicit amphetamine users. *Drug Alcohol Depend*, **48**, 235–242.

McKetin R, Mattick RP (1998) Attenton and memory in illicit amphetamine users: comparison with non-drug-using controls. *Drug Alcohol Depend*, **50**, 181–184.

MacLean MR (1999) Pulmonary hypertension, anorexigens and 5-HT: pharmacological synergism in action? *Trends Pharmacol Sci*, **20**, 490–495.

McNall M, Remafedi G (1999) Relationship of amphetamine and other substance use to unprotected intercourse among young men who have sex with men. *Arch Pediatr Adolesc Med*, **153**, 1130–1135.

Mack F, Bonisch H (1970) Dissociation constants and lipophilicity of catecholamines and related compounds. *Naunyn Schmiedebergs Arch Pharmacol*, **310**, 1–9.

Madden LJ, Flynn CT, Zanonatti MA, *et al.* (2005) Modeling human methamphetamine exposure in nonhuman primates: chronic dosing in the rhesus macaque leads to behavioral and physiological abnormalities. *Neuropsychopharmacology*, **30**, 350–359.

Magill RA, Waters WF, Bray GA, *et al.* (2003) Effects of tyrosine, phentermine, caffeine, D-amphetamine, and placebo on cognitive and motor performance deficits during sleep deprivation. *Nutr Neurosci*, **6**, 237–246.

Malay M (2001) Unintentional methamphetamine intoxication. *J Emerg Med*, **27**, 13–16.

Malberg JE, Seiden LS (1998) Small changes in ambient temperature cause large changes in 3,4-methylenedioxymethamphetamine (MDMA)-induced serotonin neurotoxicity and core body temperature in the rat. *J Neurosci*, **18**, 5086–5094.

Malchow-Møller A, Larsen S, Hey H, Stokholm KH, Juhl E, Quaade F (1981) Ephedrine as an anorectic: the story of the 'Elsinore pill'. *Int J Obes*, **5**, 183–187.

Mandell AJ (1976) *The Nightmare Season*. New York: Random House.

Mandell AJ, Stewart KD, Russo PV (1981) The Sunday syndrome: from kinetics to altered consciousness. *Fed Proc*, **40**, 2693–2698.

Manson JE, Faich GA (1996) Pharmacotherapy for obesity—do the benefits outweight the risks? [Editorial] *N Engl J Med*, **335**, 659–660.

Martin WR, Sloan JW, Sapira JD, Jasinski DR (1971) Physiologic, subjective, and behavioral effects of amphetamine, methamphetamine, ephedrine, phenmetrazine and methylphenidate in man. *Clin Pharmacol Ther*, **12**, 245–258.

Masaki T (1956) The amphetamine problem in Japan. *World Health Org Tech Rep Ser*, **102**, 14–21.

Masson J, Sagné C, Hamon M, El Mestikawy S (1999) Neurotransmitter transporters in the central nervous system. *Pharmacol Rev*, **51**, 439–464.

Mattay VS, Callicott JH, Bertolino A, *et al.* (2000) Effects of dextroamphetamine on cognitive performance and cortical activation. *NeuroImage*, **12**, 268–275.

Mattay VS, Goldberg TE, Fera F, *et al.* (2003) Catechol-O-methyltransferase val[158]-met genotype and individual variation in the brain response to amphetamine. *Proc Natl Acad Sci USA*, **100**, 6186–6191.

Matthysse S (1973) Antipsychotic drug actions: a clue to the pathology of schizophrenia? *Fed Proc*, **32**, 200–205.

Mechan AO, Esteban B, O'Shea E, Elliott JM, Colado MI, Green AR (2002) The pharmacology of the acute hyperthermic response that follows administration of 3,4-methylenedioxymethamphetamine (MDMA, 'Ecstasy'). *Br J Pharmacol*, **135**, 170–180.

Mehta MA, Sahakian BJ, Robbins TW (2001) Comparative psychopharmacology of methylphenidate and related drugs in human volunteers, patients with ADHD and experimental animals. In: Solanto MV, Arnsetein AFT, Castellanos FX (ed) *Stimulant Drugs and ADHD*. Oxford: Oxford University Press, 303–331.

Melega WP, Quintana J, Raleigh MJ, *et al.* (1996) 6-[18F]fluoro-L-DOPA–PET studies show partial reversibility of long-term effects of chronic amphetamine in monkeys. *Synapse*, **22**, 63–69.

Melega WP, Raleigh MJ, Stout DB, Yu DC, Huang SC, Phelps ME (1997) Ethological and 6-[18F]fluoro-L-DOPA-PET profiles of long-term vulnerability to chronic amphetamine. *Behav Brain Res*, **84**, 259–268.

Mennear JH (1965) Interaction between central cholinergic agents and amphetamine in mice. *Psychopharmacology*, **7**, 107–114.

Miller MA (1997) History and epidemiology of amphetamine abuse in the United States. In: Klee H (ed) *Amphetamine Misuse*. Reading, UK: Harwood Academic, 113–133.

Miller RJ, Horn AS, Iversen LL (1974) The actions of neuroleptic drugs on dopamine-stimulated adenosine cyclic 3′,5′-monophosphate production in rat neostriatum and limbic forebrain. *Mol Pharmacol*, **10**, 759–766.

Milroy CM (1999) Ten years of 'ecstasy'. *J R Soc Med*, **92**, 68–72.

Milroy CM, Clark JC, Forrest ARW (1996) The pathology of deaths associatedwith 'Eve' and 'Ecstasy' misuse. *J Clin Pathol*, **49**, 149–153.

Modell W (1960) Status and prospect of drugs for overeating. *JAMA*, **173**, 1131–1136.

Modell W, Reader GG (1970) Anorexiants. In Modell W (ed) *Drugs of Choice*. St Louis, MO: Mosby.

Molitor F, Traux CR, Ruiz JD, Sun RK (1998) Association of methamphetamine use during sex with risky sexual behaviours and HIV infection among non-injection drug users. *West J Med*, **168**, 1065–1073.

Molliver DC, Molliver ME (1990) Anatomic evidence for a neurotoxic effect of (±)fenfluramine upon serotonergic projections in the rat, *Brain Res*, **511**, 165–168.

Monroe RR, Drell HJ (1947) Oral use of stimulants obtained from inhalers. *JAMA*, **135**, 909–914.

Morgan MJ (2000) Ecstasy (MDMA): a review of its possible persistent psychological effects. *Psychopharmacology*, **152**, 230–248.

Morgan P, Beck J (1997) The legacy and the paradox: hidden contexts of methamphetamine use in the United States. In: Klee H (ed) *Amphetamine Misuse*. Reading, UK: Harwood Academic, 135–162.

Morón JA, Brockington A, Wise RA, Rocha BA, Hope BT (2002) Dopamine uptake through the norepinephrine transporter in brain regions with low levels of the dopamine transporter: evidence from knock-out mouse lines. *J Neurosci*, **22**, 389–395.

Mundy A (2001) *Dispensing with the Truth*. New York: St Martin's Press.

Murphy KR, Adler LA (2004) Assessing attention deficit hyperactivity disorder in adults: focus on rating scales. *J Clin Psychiatry*, **65** (Suppl 3), 12–17.

Murray J (1998) Psychophysiological aspects of amphetamine-methamphetamine abuse. *J Psychol*, **132**, 227–237.

Myerson A (1936) Effect of Benzedrine sulfate on mood and fatigue in normal and in neurotic persons. *Arch Neurol Psychiatry*, **36**, 816–822.

Nathanson MH (1937) The central action of beta-aminopropylbenzene (Benzedrine): clinical observations. *JAMA*, **108**, 528–531.

Nathensohn AL (1956) Clinical evaluation of Ritalin. *Dis Nerv Syst*, **17**, 394.

Neary, NM, Goldstone AP, Bloom SR (2004) Appetite regulation: from the gut to the hypothalamus. *Clin Endocrinol*, **60**, 153–160.

Necheles H, Sorter H (1957) Balanced amphetamine and sedative combination in the treatment of obesity. *Lancet*, **i**, 215–216.

Nestler EJ (2004) Molecular mechanisms of drug addiction. *Neuropharmacology*, **47**, 24–32.

Newhouse PA, Belenky G, Thomas M, Thorne D, Sing HC, Fertig J (1989) The effects of *d*-amphetamine on arousal, cognition, and mood after prolonged total sleep deprivation. *Neuropsychopharmacology*, **2**, 153–164.

Newton-Howes G (2004) What happens when children with attention deficit/hyperactivity disorder grow up? *J R Soc Med*, **97**, 531–535.

Nichols D (2001) The chemistry of MDMA. In Holland J (ed) *Ecstasy: the Complete Guide*. Rochester, VT: Park Street Press, 39–53.

Nordahl TE, Salo R, Leamon M (2003) Neuropsychological effects of chronic methamphetamine use on neurotransmitters and cognition: a review. *J Neuropsychiatry*, **15**, 317–325.

Nordstrom AL, Farde L, Ericksson L, Halldin C (1995) No elevated D_2 dopamine receptors in neuroleptic-naïve schizophrenic patients revealed by positron emission tomography and [^{11}C]N-methylspiperone. *Psychiatry Res*, **61**, 67–83.

Olds ME (1990) Enhanced dopamine receptor activation in accumbens and frontal cortex has opposite effects on medial forebrain bundle self-stimulation. *Neuroscience*, **35**, 313–325.

Olds ME, Milner P (1954) Positive reinforcement produced by electrical stimulation of septal area and other regions of rat brain. *J Comp Physiol Psychol*, **47**, 419–427.

Oswald I (1968) Drugs and sleep. *Pharmacol Rev*, **20**, 273–303.

Oswald I, Thacore VR (1963) Amphetamine and phenmetrazine addiction: physiological abnormalities in the abstinence syndrome. *BMJ*, **ii**, 427–434.

Owen F, Crow TJ, Poulter M, Cross AJ, Longden A, Riley GJ (1979) Increased dopamine-receptor sensitivity in schizophrenia. *Lancet*, **ii**, 223–225.

Parrott AC (2002) Recreational Ecstasy/MDMA, the serotonin syndrome, and serotonergic neurotxicity. *Pharmacol Biochem Behav*, **71**: 837–844.

Parrott AC (2005) Chronic tolerance to recreational MDMA (3,4-methylene-dioxymethamphetamine) or ecstasy. *J Psychopharmacol*, **19**, 71–93.

Parrott AC, Lasky J (1998) Ecstasy (MDMA) effects on mood and cognition before, during, and after a Saturday night dance. *Psychopharmacology*, **139**, 261–268.

Paulus MP, Hozack NE, Zauscher BE, *et al*. (2002) Behavioral and functional neuroimaging evidence for prefrontal dysfunction in methamphetamine-dependent subjects. *Neuropsychopharmacology*, **26**, 53–63.

Peoples SA, Guttmann E (1936) Hypertension produced with Benzedrine: its psychological accompaniments. *Lancet*, **i**, 1107–1109.

Peroutka SJ (1987) Incidence of recreational use of 3,4-methylenedioxy-amphetamine (MDMA, 'Ecstasy') on an undergraduate campus. *N Engl J Med*, **371**, 1542–1543.

Peroutka SJ, Pascoe N, Faull KF (1987) Monoamine metabolites in the cerebrospinal fluid of recreational users of 3,4-methylenedioxymethamphetamine (MDMA) ('Ecstasy'). *Res Commun Subst Abuse*, **8**, 125–138.

Peters A, Davies T, Richardson A (1997) Increasing popularity of injection as the route of administration of amphetamine in Edinburgh. *Drug Alcohol Depend*, **48**, 227–234.

Pickens R, Thompson T, Tokel RA (1972) Characteristics of amphetamine self-administration by rats. In: Ellinwood EH, Cohen S (ed) *Current Concepts on Amphetamine Abuse*. Washington, DC: US Government Printing Office, 43–48.

Piness G, Miller H, Alles GA (1930) Clinical observations on phenyl-aminoethanol sulphate *JAMA*, **94**, 790–791.

Price MTC, Fibiger HC (1974) Apomorphine and amphetamine stereotypy after 6-hydroxydopamine lesions of the substantia nigra. *Eur J Pharmacol*, **29**, 249–252.

Prinzmetal M, Bloomberg W (1935) The use of Benzedrine for the treatment of narcolepsy. *JAMA*, **105**, 2051–2054.

Randrup A, Munkvad I (1970) Biochemical, anatomical and psychological investigations of stereotyped behaviour induced by amphetamines. In: Costa E, Garratini S (ed) *Amphetamine and Related Compounds*. New York: Raven Press, 695–713.

Randrup A, Munkvad I (1974) Pharmacology and physiology of stereotyped behaviour. *J Psychiatr Res*, **11**, 1–10.

Rapoport JL, Buchsbaum MS, Weingartner H, Zahn TP, Ludlow C (1980). Dextroamphetamine: cognitive and behavioral effects in normal and hyperactive boys and normal men. *Arch Gen Psychiatry*, **37**, 933.

Rapport MD, Carlson GA, Kelly KL, Pataki C (1993) Methylphenidate and desipramine in hospitalized children: I. Separate and combined effects on cognitive function. *J Am Acad Child Adolesc Psychiatry*, **32**, 333–342.

Rawson R, Shoptaw S, Obert JL, *et al.* (1995) An intensive outpatient approach for cocaine abuse: the Matrix model. *J Subst Abuse Treat* **12**, 117–127.

Rawson R, Huber A, Brethen P, *et al.* (2000) Methamphetamine and cocaine users: differences in characteristics and treatment retention. *J Psychoactive Drugs*, **32**, 233–238.

Rawson RA, Marinelli-Casey P, Anglin MD, Dickow A, Frazier Y, Gallagher C, Galloway GP, Herrell J, Huber A, McCann MJ, Obert J, Pennell S, Reiber C, Vandersloot D, Zweben J (2004) Methamphetamine Treatment Project Corporate Authors. A multi-site comparison of psychosocial approaches for the treatment of methamphetamine dependence. *Addiction*. **99**, 708-717.

Rechtschaffen A, Maron L (1964) The effect of amphetamine on the sleep cycle. *Electoencephalogr Clin Neurophysiol*, **16**, 438–445.

Reifenstein EC Jr, Davidoff E (1939) Benzedrine sulfate therapy: the present status. *NY State J Med*, **39**, 42–57.

Reneman L, Booij J, de Bruin K, *et al*. (2001) Effects of dose, sex, and long term abstention from use on toxic effects of MDMA (ecstasy) on brain serotonin neurons. *Lancet*, **358**, 1864–1869.

Reynolds S (1998) *Energy Flash: A Journey Through Rave Music and Dance Culture*. London: Picador.

Ricaurte GA, Yuan J, McCann UD (2000) ($\pm$)3,4-Methylenedioxy-methamphetamine ('Ecstasy')-induced serotonin neurotoxicity: studies in animals. *Neuropsychobiology*, **42**, 5–10.

Ricaurte GA, Yuan J, Hatzidimitriou G, Cord BJ, McCann UD (2002) Severe dopaminergic neurotoxicity in primates after a single recreational dose regimen of MDMA ('Ecstasy'). *Science*, **297**, 2260–2263.

Ricaurte GA, Yuan J, Hatzidimitiou G, Cord BJ, McCann US (2003) Retraction. *Science*, **301**, 1479.

Robbins TW (2002) The 5-choice serial reaction time task: behavioural pharmacology and functional neurochemistry. *Psychopharmacology*, **163**, 362–380.

Robbins TW, Sahakian BJ (1979) Paradoxical effects of psychomotor stimulant drugs in hyperactive children from the standpoint of behavioural pharmacology. *Neuropharmacology*, **18**, 931–950.

Robin AA, Weisberg S (1958) A controlled trial of methyl phenidate (Ritalin) in the treatment of depressive states. *J Neurol Neurosurg Psychiatry*, **21**, 57.

Robson P, Bruce M (1997) A comparison of 'visible' and 'invisible' users of amphetamine, cocaine and heroin: two distinct populations. *Addiction*, **92**, 1729–1736.

Rothman RB, Baumann MH (2003) Monoamine transporters and psychostimulant drugs. *Eur J Pharmacol*, **479**, 23–40.

Rutter M, Cox A, Tupling C, Berger M, Yule W (1975) Attainment and adjustment in two geographical areas. I: The prevalence of psychiatric disorders. *Br J Psychiatry*, **126**, 493–509.

Rylander G (1969) Clinical and medico-criminological aspects of addiction to central stimulating drugs. In: Sjoqvist F, Tottie M (ed) *Abuse of Control Stimulants*. Stockholm: Almqvist and Wiksell, 251–273.

Rylander G (1971) Stereotype behaviour in man following amphetamine abuse. In: Baker SB deC (ed) *The Correlation of Adverse Effects in Man with Observations in Animals*. Amsterdam: Excerpta Medica, 28–31.

Sadusk JR (1966) Non-narcotic addiction: size and extent of the problem. *JAMA*, **196**, 707–709.

Salo R, Nordahl TE, Possin K, *et al.* (2002) Preliminary evidence of reduced cognitive inhibition in methamphetamine-dependent individuals. *Psychiatry Res*, **111**, 65–74.

Samaha AN, Robinson TE (2005) Why does the rapid delivery of drugs to the brain promote addiction? *Trends Pharmacol Sci*, **26**, 82–87.

Sanello F (2005) *Tweakers: How Crystal Meth is Ravaging Gay America*. Los Angeles, CA: Alyson.

Sannerud C, Feussner G (2000) Is Ritalin an abused drug? Does it meet the criteria of a Schedule II substance? In: Greenhill LL, Osman BB (ed) *Ritalin, Theory and Practice*. New Rochelle, NY: Mary Ann Liebert, 27–44.

Sannerud CA, Brady JV, Griffiths RR (1989) Self-injection in baboons of amphetamines and related designer drugs. *NIDA Res Monogr*, **94**, 30–42.

Sargent W, Blackburn JM (1936) The effect of Benzedrine on intelligence scores. *Lancet*, **ii**, 1385–1387.

Saunders M (1997) *Ecstasy Reconsidered*. London: Nicholas Saunders.

Scheffel U, Lever JR, Mathews WB, *et al.* (1998) *In vivo* detection of short and long-term MDMA neurotoxicity–a positron emission tomography study in the living baboon brain. *Synapse*, **29**, 183–192.

Schifano F, Oyefeso A, Webb L, Pollar M, Corkery J, Ghodse AH (2003) Review of deaths related to taking ecstasy, England and Wales, 1997–2002. *BMJ*, **326**, 80–81.

Schindler CW, Zheng JW, Tella SR, Goldberg SR (1992) Pharmacological mechanisms in the cardiovascular effects of methamphetamine in conscious squirrel monkeys. *Pharmacol Biochem Behav*, **42**, 791–796.

Schliefer J (1998) *Methamphetamines: Speed Kills*. New York: Rosen.

Schuster CR, Woods JH, Seevers MH (1969) Self-administration of control stimulants by the monkey. In: Sjoqvist F, Tottie M (ed) *Abuse of Control Stimulants*. Stockholm: Almqvist and Wiksell, 339–347.

Scott MS (2003) *Clandestine Drug Labs. Problem Oriented Guide for Police Series No 16*. Washington, DC: US Department of Justice.

Sedvall G (1975) Receptor feedback and dopamine turnover in CNS. In: Iversen LL, Iversen SD, Snyder SH (ed) *Handbook of Psychopharmacology*, Vol 6. New York: Plenum Press, 127–177.

Sedvall G, Fyro B, Nyback H, Wiesel FA (1975) Actions of dopaminergic antagonists in the striatum. *Adv Neurol*, **9**, 131–140.

Seeman P, Kapur S (2000) Commentary: 'Schizophrenia: more dopamine, more D_2 receptors'. *Proc Natl Acad Sci USA*, **97**, 7673–7675.

Seeman P, Chau-Wong M, Tedesco J, Wong K (1975) Brain receptors for antipsychotic drugs and dopamine: direct binding assays. *Proc Natl Acad Sci USA*, **72**, 4376–4380.

Seeman P, Titeler M, Tedesco J, Weinreich P, Sinclair D (1978) Brain receptors for dopamine and neuroleptics. *Adv Biochem Psychopharmacol*, **19**, 167–176.

Seeman P, Weinshenker D, Quirion R, *et al.* (2005) Dopamine supersensitivity correlates with D2High states, implying many paths to psychosis. *Proc Natl Acad Sci USA*, **102**, 3513–3518.

Segal DS, Kuczenski R (1992) *In vivo* microdialysis reveals a diminished amphetamine-induced dopamine response corresponding to behavioral sensitization produced by repeated amphetamine pretreatment. *Brain Res*, **571**, 330–337.

Segal DS, Kuczenski R (1996) Behavioral pharmacology of amphetamine. In: Cho AK, Segal DS (ed) *Amphetamine and its Analogs: Neuropharmacology, Toxicology and Abuse*. New York: Academic Press, 115–149.

Segal DS, Kuczenski R, O'Neil ML, Melega WP, Cho AK (2003) Escalating dose methamphetamine pretreatment alters the behavioral and neurochemical profiles associated with exposure to a high-dose methamphetamine binge. *Neuropsychopharmacology*, **28**, 1730–1740.

Seghatol FF, Rigolin VH (2002) Appetite suppressants and valvular heart disease. *Curr Opin Cardiol*, **17**, 486–492.

Seiden LS, Fischman MW, Schuster CR (1976) Long-term methamphetamine induced changes in brain catecholamines in tolerant rhesus monkeys. *Drug Alcohol Depend*, **1**, 215–219.

Seiden LS, Sabol KE, Ricaurte GA (1993) Amphetamine effects on catecholamine systems and behavior. *Annu Rev Pharmacol Toxicol*, **33**, 639–677.

Sekine Y, Minabe Y, Ouchi Y, *et al.* (2003) Association of dopamine transporter loss in the orbitofrontal and dorsolateral prefrontal cortices with methamphetamine-related psychiatric symptoms. *Am J Psychiatry*, **160**, 1699–1701.

Select Committee on Crime (1971) *Amphetamines*. 91st Congress, 2nd Session, House Report No 91–1807. Washington, DC: US Government Printing Office.

Semple DH, Ebmeier KP, Glabus MF, O'Carroll RE, Johnstone EC (1999) Reduced *in vivo* binding to the serotonin transporter in the cerebral cortex of MDMA ('ecstasy') users. *Br J Psychiatry*, **175**, 63–69.

Semple SJ, Patterson TL, Grant I (2002) Motivations associated with methamphetamine use among HIV+ men who have sex with men. J Subst Abuse Treat, **22**, 149–156.

Sesack SR, Hawrylak VA, Matus C, Guido MA, Levey AL (1998) Dopamine axon varicosities in the prelimbic division of the rat prefrontal cortex exhibit sparse immunoreactivity for the dopamine transporter. *J Neurosci*, **18**, 2697–2708.

Setola V, Hufeisen SJ, Grande-Allen J, *et al.* (2003) 3,4-Methylene-dioxymethamphetamine (MDMA, 'Ecstasy') induces fenfluramine-like proliferative actions on human cardiac valvular interstitial cells *in vitro*. *Mol Pharmacol*, **63**, 1223–1229.

Shapiro RP, Michaile KJ (1956) The use of a sustained-release *d*-amphetamine-amobarbital preparation in the treatment of obesity. *Int Rec Med Gen Pract Clin*, **169**, 638–641.

Shearer J, Wodak A, Mattick RP, Lewis J, Hall W, Dolan K (2001) Pilot randomized controlled study of dexamphetamine substitution for amphetamine dependence. *Addiction*, **96**, 1289–1296.

Shoblock JR, Sullivan EB, Maisonneuve IM, Glick S (2003) Neurochemical and behavioral differences between *d*-methamphetamine and *d*-amphetamine in rats. *Psychopharmacology*, **165**, 359–369.

Shulgin AT (1986) The background and chemistry of MDMA. *J Psychoactive Drugs*, **18**, 291–304.

Shulgin A, Shulgin A (2000) *PIHKAL: A Chemical Love Story*. Berkeley, CA: Transform Press.

Silverstone T (1992) Appetite suppressants: a review. *Drugs*, **43**, 820–836.

Simon SL, Domier C, Carnell J, Brethen P, Rawson L, Ling W (2000) Cognitive impairment in individuals currently using methamphetamine. *Am J Addict*, **9**, 222–231.

Simon SL, Dacey J, Glynn S, Rawson R, Ling W (2004) The effect of relapse on cognition in abstinent methamphetamine abusers. *J Subst Abuse Treat*, **27**, 59–66.

Smith DE, Fischer CM (1970) An analysis of 310 cases of acute high-dose methamphetamine toxicity in Haight-Ashbury. *Clin Toxicol*, **3**, 117–124.

Smith GM, Beecher HK (1959) Amphetamine sulfate and athletic performance. I: Objective effects. *JAMA*, **170**, 542–557.

Snyder SH (1972) Catecholamines in the brain as mediators of amphetamine psychosis. *Arch Gen Psychiatry*, **27**, 169–179.

Snyder SH, Banerjee SP, Yamamura HI, Greenberg D (1974) Drugs, neurotransmitters and schizophrenia. *Science*, **184**, 1243–1245.

Solanto MV (1986) Behavioral effects of low-dose methylphenidate in childhood attention deficit disorder: implications for a mechanism of stimulant drug action. *J Am Acad Child Adolesc Psychiatry*, **25**, 96–101.

Solanto MV (1998) Neuropsychopharmacological mechanism of stimulant drug action in attention-deficit hyperactivity disorder: a review and integration. *Behav Brain Res*, **94**, 127–152.

Solanto MV, Arnstein AFT and Castellanos FX (2001) The neuroscience of stimulant drug action in ADHD. In: Solanto MV, Arnsetein AFT, Castellanos FX (ed) *Stimulant Drugs and ADHD*. Oxford: Oxford University Press, 355–379.

Sotelo C (1991) Immunohistochemical study of short- and long-term effects of *d, l*-fenfluramine on the serotonergic innervation of the rat hippocampal formation. *Brain Res*, **541**, 309–326.

Spencer T, Biederman J, Wilens T (2004) Stimulant treatment of adult attention deficit/hyperactivity disorder. *Psychiatr Clin N Am*, **27**,361–372.

Srisurapanont M, Jarusuraisin N, Kittirattanapaiboon P (2003) Treatment for amphetamine dependence and abuse (Cochrane Review). In: *The Cochrane Library*. Chichester: John Wiley and Sons.

Stefanski R, Ladenheim B, Lee SH, Cadet JL, Goldberg SR (1999) Neuroadaptations in the dopaminergic system after active self-administration but not after passive administration of methamphetamine. *Eur J Pharmacol*, **371**, 123–135.

Stefanski R, Lee SH, Cadet JL, Goldberg SR (2002) Lack of persistent changes in the dopaminergic system of rats withdrawn from methamphetamine self-administration. *Eur J Pharmacol*, **439**, 59–68.

Stein MA, Waldman I, Sarampote C, Seymour K, Robb A, Conlon C (2002) Dopamine transporter genotype (DAT1) affects stimulant response in children with ADHD. *Am J Hum Genet*, **18**, 420–425.

Steinkamp P (2003) Pervitin (metamphetamine) experiments and its use in the German Wehrmacht. http://www.geschichte.uni-freiburg.de/DFG-Geschichte/MedTagungAbstracts.htm

Still GF (1902) Some abnormal psychical conditions in children. *Lancet*, **i**, 1008–1012.

Strakowski SM, Sax KW, Setters MJ, Keck PE Jr (1996) *Biol Psychiatry*, **40**, 872–880.

Sumnall HR, Cole JC (2005) Self-reported depressive symptomatology in community samples of polysubstance misusers who report Ecstasy use: a meta-analysis. *J. Psychopharmacol*, **19**, 84–92.

Suwaki H (1991) Methamphetamine abuse in Japan. *NIDA Res Monogr*, **115**, 84–96.

Swanson JM, Volkow ND (2001) Pharmacokinetic and pharmacodynamic properties of methylphenidate in humans. In: Solanto MV, Arnsetein AFT, Castellanos FX (ed) *Stimulant Drugs and ADHD*. Oxford: Oxford University Press, 259–282.

Swanson JM, Volkow ND (2003) Serum and brain concentrations of methylphenidate: implications for use and abuse. *Neurosci Biobehav Rev*, **27**, 615–621.

Szuster RR (1990) Methamphetamine in psychiatric emergencies. *Hawaii Med*, **49**, 389–391.

Tamblyn R, Berkson L, Jauphine WD, *et al*. (1996) Unnecessary prescribing of NSAIDs and the management of NSAID-related gastropathy in medical practice. *Ann Int Med*, **127**, 429–438.

Tatetsu S (1964) Methamphetamine psychosis. *Folia Psychiatr Neurol Jpn*, **7** (Suppl), 377–380.

Thal N (1969) Cumulative index of antidepressant medications. *Dis Nerv Syst*, **20**, 201.

Thim L, Kristensen P, Larsen PJ, Wulff BS (1998) CART, a new anorectic peptide. *Int J Biochem Cell Biol*, **30**, 1281–1284.

Thompson HS (1967) *The Hell's Angels*. New York: Ballantine.

Thompson PM, Hayashi KM, Simon SL, *et al*. (2004) Structural abnormalities in the brain of human subjects who use methamphetamine. *J Neurosci*, **24**, 6028–6036.

Thornburg JE, Moore KE (1973) The relative importance of dopaminergic and noradrenergic neuronal systems for the stimulation of locomotor activity induced by amphetamine and other drugs. *Neuropharmacology*, **12**, 853–866.

Tinklenberg JR, Stillman RC (1970) Drug use and violence. In: Daniels DN, Gilula MF, Ochberg FM (ed) *Violence and the Struggle for Existence*. Boston, MA: Little Brown, 335–336.

Turner JJD, Parrott AC (2000) Is MDMA a human neurotoxin? Diverse views from the discussants. *Neuropsychobiology*, **42**, 42–48.

Trendelenburg U (1963) Mechanisms of supersensitivity and subsensitivity to sympathomimetic amines. *Pharmacol Rev*, **15**, 225–276.

Trendelenburg U (1991) Functional aspects of the uptake of noradrenaline. *Trends Pharmacol Sci*, **12**, 334–337.

Tyler DB (1947) The effect of amphetamine sulfate and some barbiturates on the fatigue produced by prolonged wakefulness. *Am J Physiol*, **150**, 253–262.

Tzschentke TM, Schmidt WJ (2000) Functional relationship among medial prefrontal cortex, nucleus accumbens, and ventral tegmental area in locomotion and reward. *Crit Rev Neurobiol*, **14**, 131–142.

Ungless MA (2004) Dopamine: the salient issue. *Trends Neurosci*, **27**, 702–706.

United Nations (2003) Ecstasy and amphetamines—global survey. [http://www.unodc.org/pdf/publications/report_ats_2003.09.23_1.pdf]

United Nations (2005) World Drug Report 2005 [www.unodc.org/pdf/WDR_2005/volume_2_chap8_drugabuse.pdf]

Van Kammen DP, Bunney WE Jr (1982) Testing the dopamine hypothesis of schizophrenia: response to *d*-amphetamine and pimozide. In Namba M, Kaiya H (ed) *Psychobiology of Schizophrenia*. Oxford: Pergamon Press, 265–275.

Van Kammen DP, Bunney WE Jr, Docherty JP, *et al.* (1982) *d*-Amphetamine-induced heterogeneous changes in psychotic behaviour in schizophrenia. *Am J Psychiatry*, **139**, 991–997.

Verducci T (2002) Getting amped. *Sports Illustrated*, **96**, 23.

Voet W (2002) *Breaking the Chain* (trans W. Fotheringham). London: Yellow Jersey Press.

Volkow ND (2005) Methamphetamine abuse. http://www.nida.nih.gov/Testimony/4–21–05Testimony.html

Volkow ND, Li TK (2004) Drug addiction: the neurobiology of behaviour gone awry. *Nat Rev Neurosci*, **5**, 963–970.

Volkow ND, Wang GJ, Fowler JS, *et al.* (1999) Methylphenidate and cocaine have a similar *in vivo* potency to block dopamine transporters in the human brain. *Life Sci*, **65**, PL7–12.

Volkow ND, Chang L, Wang GJ, *et al.* (2001) Higher cortical and lower sub-cortical metabolism in detoxified methamphetamine abusers. *Am J Psychol*, **158**, 383–389.

Volkow ND, Wang GF, Fowler JS, *et al.* (2003) Brain DA D2 receptors predict reinforcing effects of stimulants in humans: replication study. *Synapse*, **46**, 79–82.

Volkow ND, Wang GJ, Fowler JS, *et al.* (2004) Evidence that methylphenidate enhances the saliency of a mathematical task by increasing dopamine in the human brain. *Am J Psychiatry*, **161**, 1173–1180.

Völlm BA, de Araujo IE, Cowen PJ, *et al.* (2004) Methamphetamine activates reward circuitry in drug naïve human subjects. *Neuropsychopharmacology*, **29**, 1715–1722.

Wallach MB (1974) Drug-induced stereotyped behaviour: similarities and differences. In: Usdin E (ed) *Neuropsychopharmacology of Monoamines and their Regulatory Enzymes*. New York: Raven Press, 241–260.

Wang GJ, Volkow ND, Chang L, *et al.* (2004) Partial recovery of brain metabolism in methamphetamine abusers after protracted abstinence. *Am J Psychiatry*, **161**, 242–248.

Ward MF, Wender LH, Reinherr FW (1993) The Wender Utah Rating Scale: an aid to the retrospective diagnosis of childhood attention deficit hyperactivity disorder. *Am J Psychiatry*, **150**, 885–890.

Waud SP (1938) The effects of toxic doses of benzyl methyl carbinamine (Benzedrine) in man. *JAMA*, **110**, 206–207.

Weintraub M (1992) Long term weight control study: conclusions. *Clin Pharmacol Ther*, **51**, 642–646.

Weir EK, Reeve HL, Huang JMC, *et al.* (1996) Experimental myocardial ischemia/myocardial infarction/pulmonary artery constriction: anorexic agents aminorex, fenfluramine, and dexfenfluramine inhibit potassium current in rat pulmonary vascular smooth muscle and cause pulmonary vasoconstriction. *Circulation*, **94**, 2216–2220.

Weiss B, Laties VG (1962) Enhancement of human performance by caffeine and the amphetamines. *Pharmacol Rev*, **14**, 1–36.

Weissman A, Koe BK, Tenen SS (1966) Antiamphetamine effects following inhibition of tyrosine hydroxylase. *J Pharmacol Exp Ther*, **151**, 329–352.

Wellman PJ, Maher TJ (1999) Synergistic interactions between fenfluramine and phentermine. *Int J Obes*, **23**, 723–732

Wender PH (2001) *ADHD: Attention-Deficit Hyperactivity Disorder in Children, Adolescents and Adults*. New York: Oxford University Press.

Wheatley D (1969) Amphetamines in general practice: their use in depression and anxiety. *Semin Psychiatry*, **1**, 163–173.

White TL, Justice AJH, de Wit H (2002) Differential subjective effects of D-amphetamine by gender, hormone levels and menstrual cycle phase. *Pharmacol Biochem Behav*, **73**, 729–741.

WHO Expert Committee on Addiction-Producing Drugs (1964) Thirteenth Report. *WHO Tech Rep Ser*, **273**, 9–10.

Wigal SB, McGough JJ, McCracken JT, Biederman J, Spencer TJ, Posner KL, Wigal TL, Kollins SH, Clark TM, Mays DA, Zhansg Y, Tulloch SJ (2005)

A laboratory school comparison of mixed amphetamine salts extended release (Adderall XR) and atomoxetine (Strattera) in school-aged children with attention deficit/hyperactivity disorder. *J Atten Disord*, **9**, 275-289.

Wilens TE, Biederman J, Spencer TJ (2002) Attention deficit/hyperactivity disorder across the lifespan. *Annu Rev Med*, **53**, 113–131.

Wilens TE, Faraone SV, Biederman J, Dunawardene S (2003) Does stimulant therapy of attention-deficit/hyperactivity disorder beget later substance abuse? A meta-analytic review of the literature. *Pediatrics*, **111**, 179–185.

Wilson JM, Kalasinsky KS, Levey AI, *et al.* (1996) Striatal dopamine nerve terminal markers in human, chronic methamphetamine users. *Nat Med*, **2**, 699–703.

Wolraich ML, Doffing MA (2004) Pharmacokinetic considerations in the treatment of attention-deficit hyperactivity disorder with methylphenidate. *CNS Drugs*, **18**, 243–250.

Wong DF, Pearlson GD, Tune LE, *et al.* (1997) *Quantification of neuroreceptors in the living human brain. IV: Effect of aging and elevations of D2-like receptors in schizophrenia and bipolar illness. J Cereb Blood Flow Metab*, **17**, 331–342.

Woolverton WL, Ricaurte GA, Forno LS, Seiden LS (1989) Long-term effects of chronic methamphetamine administration in rhesus monkeys. *Brain Res*, **486**, 73–78.

Wurtman J, Wurtman R, Reynolds S, Tsay R, Chew B (1987) Fenfluramine suppresses snack intake among carbohydrate cravers but not among non-carbohydrate cravers. *Int J Eat Disord*, **6**, 687–699.

Young D, Scoville WB (1938) Paranoid psychosis in narcolepsy, and the possible danger of Benzedrine treatment. *Med Clin N Am*, **22**, 637–646.

Yu Q, Larson DF, Watson RR (2003) Heart disease, methamphetamine and AIDS. *Life Sci*, **73**, 129–140.

Zahniser NR, Sorkin A (2004) Rapid regulation of the dopamine transporter: role in stimulant addiction? *Neuropharmacology*, **47**, 80–91.

Author Index

Subject Index